Fat, Fatigued & Frustrated?

How to Reverse the Clock & Feel Young Again

Glen Depke, Traditional Naturopath

Unstoppable Wellness Publishing USA

Fat, Fatigued and Frustrated? How to Reverse the Clock and Feel Young Again.

Published by Unstoppable Wellness Publishing

ISBN: 978-0-9975088-1-9

Printed in the United States of America

10 9 8 7 6 5 4 3 2 1

Dedication

I'd like to thank everyone who helped me create this book. My amazing wife Dawn for her inspiration and countless hours of editing and making this an enjoyable read for all of us. Sue Ingebretson for her professional editing expertise. Dr. Bill Janeshak for his input on Chiropractic care. And lastly, Michael Stevenson for pushing me at the onset to create this reality. Together, we put together a rockin' expression of health!

Contents

Forward

I first met Glen over a decade ago and was fascinated to learn all the work he was at the forefront of that correlated lab testing with nutritional typing. The team he was leading were years ahead in applying natural medicine concepts to people with complex health problems.

Fast forward to today. Glen continues to be a leader in the field of natural health. Now, with his new book he highlights time tested solutions to the dilemma most of us find ourselves in regarding chronic health problems. You can apply these solutions immediately to start your journey back to physical health and bring a sense of abundance and joy we are all sadly missing.

I was also a client of Glen's many years ago and he taught me the connections between our emotional health and physical well-being. Most of us have suffered from a health problem, sought out conventional medical care, been poked, prodded and tested only to be told there's nothing really wrong and that it's "all in your head." Well, it turns out that may be partially true. In functional medicine we set the stage for physical recovery by doing sophisticated lab testing not practiced in conventional medicine. These tests, such as adrenal stress tests and specialized GI testing enables practitioners the ability to offer treatments for the physical body that would be glossed over in a conventional medical work up. We also place a huge emphasis on lifestyle changes, as described in this book, sleep, exercise and a big focus on food. Ultimately once the physical body is working properly, we then need to confront the thoughts and feelings and spiritual disconnection that come with poor health.

Once your functional medicine tests are all clear and you have your diet, exercise and sleep patterns all sorted out, you'll regain a sense of physical health.

But then what? What you do with that new found sense of health makes all the difference.

I have a patient, Jonathan, an entrepreneur who retired at age 40 with over $10 million in the bank and homes in both California and Hawaii. He worked with me for two years to overcome the decades of stress and neglect that had come from his career focused life. He began sleeping perfectly, exercising perfecting, ate bite for bite perfectly, was physically in great shape. Yet after all this near obsessive focus on his recovery he was still unhappy. Even with all the money and the homes he was unsatisfied with life. Jonathan taught me that perfect health without emotional connection has little value.

This is a key example that having an emotional and spiritual connection and growth is a key component to having a satisfying life.

Another couple I work with, Brett and Sue. Sue has a serious autoimmune illness and is unable to move by herself. Brett cares for her full time, waking every 90 minutes night after night to move her into a new sleeping position. They are one of the happiest couples I've ever worked with. They are happy individuals and together their lives mesh flawlessly. Sue and Brett demonstrated to me that even in the presence of serious illness love and connection are possible to maintain.

Now most of us don't have $10 million or a life destroying autoimmune illness. Most of us have regular lives and regular problems. However most of us are emotionally and spiritually disconnected and challenged to experience the full range of human experience. We rarely have a sense of complete connection with the world and ourselves, more often experiencing the blocks in life that prevent us from the timeless, abundant and limitless universe surrounding us.

We often think if I just had X million dollars then all these problems would vanish. I know from on my own health problems in the past how hard it is to feel enlightened and spiritually aware when I was sick and not feeling good physically.

So regardless of how much money you have or don't have or what your health problems are I believe we can benefit the most from our gains in physical health if we invest them in emotional and spiritual growth.

When you begin to eat better and your energy increases from your new diet, put that energy into meditation or prayer and fully grow your spiritual life. If you start to exercise and feel more alert and less stressed fill that space with emotional balancing work to uncover and release old wounds you are still holding onto. If you start an adrenal healing program based on a functional medicine model and it works, don't just use the new found energy to feel better internally, use that internal sense of well-being to connect deeply with other people in your life.

Glen Depke

Through personal development, releasing old emotional experiences we continue to lug around and by supporting others we can truly regain our whole selves and experience day to day a sense of wonder, joy, relaxation and love that makes being on this planet worthwhile.

Glen will help you achieve this with "Fat, Fatigued & Frustrated?"

Daniel Kalish

Dr. Daniel Kalish D.C.
Founder of the Kalish Institute

Author of:
Your Guide to Healthy Hormones

The Kalish Method: Healing the Body, Mapping the Mind

About the Author

I experienced a health breakdown at the age of 17 when I felt like I was run over by a Mack truck after having my first grand mal seizure. Little did I know that this was the beginning of a healing journey and a path that would lead me to change my 20 year career and find my true passion in life.

I had every conventional medical test known to man and there was no clear or obvious reason for my seizures, so the answer was, "here, take this pill." My seizures continued for nearly a decade after religiously taking the prescription medication that was supposed to control them. Not only did the medication not work, it left me feeling fatigued and mentally confused. Another frightening side effect was decreased muscle control and coordination. I also experienced repeated sprained ankles, swollen and bleeding gums, physical pain, weight gain, and disturbances in my sleep patterns. At this point conventional medicine could not give me ONE reason for the onset nor the continuation of these seizures. Their only answer was to diagnose me as an epileptic.

I didn't know what to do. There were no answers as the plaguing symptoms and intense seizures continued. It was such an exhausting experience. I felt hopeless. My health was deteriorating and I had no guidance. I became frustrated … and that frustration turned into anger.

Feeling backed into a corner, I finally took matters into my own hands. I began researching the dangers of prescription medications. This one side effect of my main drug stood out to me like a red flag. The label insert itself said there was potential for further neurological damage!

Let me be clear, a seizure disorder is already a neurological dysfunction, so why would I want the potential to *increase* this dysfunction further? This was the turning point for me.

When I discovered the underlying causes of grand mal seizures, I took action. I removed my mercury amalgams (silver fillings), reached out for professional assistance with detoxification protocols, and changed my lifestyle habits completely. It was then that I became a patient of Dr. Joseph Mercola. Under the guidance of him and his team, I weaned myself off the seizure medication, made significant dietary and lifestyle changes, began an intense detox program, and implemented stress-release techniques.

I was able to overcome epilepsy naturally and in the process a passion erupted inside of me to assist others with healing their "incurable" health "dis-eases."

This was when my formal education began.

I am now a Traditional Naturopath and I LOVE my work!

"Naturopathy" is a hybrid term with Latin and Greek roots meaning "to benefit from Nature."

As a Traditional Naturopath I teach people how to initiate their body's own natural healing ability. Basic protocols include proper breathing and hydration, dietary improvements, movement, proper rest, sunshine, emotional release, supplement and herbal/homeopathic remedies and many other natural healing therapies.

As a Traditional Naturopath I do not "diagnose" or "treat diseases," but rather assess the whole body and recognize that the majority of health challenges are cumulative lifestyle choices such as improper diet, unhealthy habits, high levels of stress and environmental factors which lead to weakening the bodies' natural defense. Combined, these result in a breakdown in health.

My life's passion has led me to continue my education and I've become a lifelong learner. I have since earned a diploma in Professional Holistic Iridology, have become a certified Metabolic Typing advisor (customized nutrition), an emotional freedom technique (EFT) practitioner, and am trained to use traditional Chinese assessment tools as well as German drainage therapy.

I was asked to join Dr. Joseph Mercola's team at his Natural Health Center in Chicago, Illinois and eventually became his chief Nutritionist and Wellness Director. I learned cutting edge healing protocols such as The Kalish Method of Functional Medicine and have developed expertise in the areas of adrenal function, natural hormone balancing, the gut/brain connection, immune regulation and healing chronic inflammatory states.

In 2001, I founded Depke Wellness with the intention of wellness for the world. In 2008 I moved across the country and opened the Depke Wellness Holistic Healing Center located in Costa Mesa, California where I currently lead a team of experts, helping people feel young again.

We lead programs, lecture around the country, and provide on-line courses as well as working one on one with clients in our health center. We recognize the whole body. This means the physical body, the mental/emotional body, the chemical body, and your spiritual/vibrational body. We focus on understanding the underlying triggers and causes of your health challenges and balance them naturally and safely. ***This truly holistic approach enables us to get to the core of your health challenges rather than simply addressing symptoms.***

This book is a result of my research, experience, and the learnings I received from helping thousands of people, just like you, overcome varying health challenges. It's the basis for all healing and gives you a simple step by step process to kick start your healing from the inside.

This book is for those ready to take their health to the next level. I trust you'll enjoy.

Introduction

Are you feeling overweight, fatigued and frustrated? You've tried everything only to fail and you're losing hope. You want to feel young again but don't know how to reverse the clock. Take a moment and imagine what your life would look like if you never changed anything from this day forward.

Can you remember the last time you were at your ideal weight and could easily slide into your "skinny jeans?" Or how about a time when you didn't have to reach for the coffee or snacks to get you through the rest of the day? Have you ever experienced a time in your life when you were truly happy and life was effortless?

What if I gave you the secrets to get you back in your skinny jeans and look and feel young again? What if I could reveal to you, your body's innate intelligence that can guide you to feel confident, vibrant, and empowered?

You'd be interested, wouldn't you?

I know you would because I've been exactly where you are.

I felt the guilt for allowing myself to get that bad. I remember the lack of energy and trying every quick fix just to get through the day. I felt the endless frustration from knowing that nothing was working!

After years of trying different diets, exercising too little or too much, starving myself with minimal results, I finally discovered the secret to overcoming the real problem. I got back to my ideal weight and have stayed there. I also enjoy a high level energy throughout the day, feel happy, and even attractive again.

I know this is what you want, too. You want to reach your ideal weight, be energized, and feel attractive again. Of course you do ... or you wouldn't have picked up this book in the first place!

In this book I reveal proven and effective SECRETS that have not only helped me but have also helped thousands of people just like you. I outline a step by step process for you to easily reach your goals. All that's required of you is that you follow the steps, be coachable, and stay committed.

Imagine opening your closet doors and feeling as if you own twice as many clothes because EVERYTHING fits perfectly? How much happier will you be when you have energy at the end of the day, *every day?* Imagine how life feels inside your body when you're your ideal weight, are a picture of health and vitality, and feel attractive -- for the rest of your life?

Now *that* is something to think about.

"Fat, Fatigued & Frustrated?" will provide you the ability to get your life back on many levels. It's a book that helps you understand the how and why you became overweight, fatigued and frustrated in the first place. All while providing you simple, effective, and proven strategies that

will guide you to reaching your ideal weight as well as your energetic and happy self again.

Yes, I can help you reverse the clock!

Chapter One

How to Reverse the Clock and Feel Young Again

The first step in this process is to look at your **fundamentals of health.** These are the simple daily behaviors that propel you forward in reaching your ideal weight, having ample amounts of energy, aging well, attaining health from the inside out, and allowing you to experience happiness and fulfillment at deep levels.

The Depke Wellness Fundamentals of Health Include:

- The air you breathe
- The water you drink
- The food you eat
- The quality of your sleep
- Movement
- Exposure to the sun

- Mental, emotional, spiritual, and energetic health
- Bonus Section: Deeper healing

Imagine the following type of life. Imagine putting your head on the pillow and immediately falling into a deep sleep. Upon waking you feel rested, energized, and excited for the start of your new day. At each meal, your food choices are healthy. Your body feels completely satisfied with sustained energy to last throughout the entire day. Your mental clarity increases and you're finding situations that were once stressful, are now much easier to handle.

You feel yourself naturally taking deep breathes throughout the day. This helps you feel more grounded and peaceful. You hear your colleagues and friends asking what you're doing because you look fabulous and they want to do what you're doing.

You feel a deep joy that you have never felt before. A sense of calm and confidence has replaced the stress and frustration that used to be commonplace. You have more motivation, a sense of empowerment, and feel in control and inspired.

Life has gone from effort and struggle to daily ease.

Once you begin to make these small consistent changes in your fundamentals of health, the scenarios listed above are possible. These are the results I hear time and time again from the people I help.

You are no different.

It's no coincidence that you're reading this book right now. You are ready for change and I'm going to give you the process to make that happen.

Let's begin!

The Air You Breathe

You might be thinking, "I'm living so I am breathing, right?"

Yes, but the question I invite you to ask yourself is, "Am I breathing to survive or I am breathing to thrive?" There's a significant difference between the two.

Most of us live very busy stressful lives. This leaves us in what I call a "defensive posture." You've seen many people in this scenario and possibly experienced it yourself at times. You simply didn't recognize it. This is how it looks. Whether standing or sitting, the shoulders are rounded forward with the chest caving in a bit. There's a little slump in the back. This compromised posture is the body's natural response as a form of protection from our busy stressful lives. The combination of the stress and this "forced" posture leaves us taking short, shallow breathes through the day. This unnatural breathing pattern is insufficient for optimal health.

Go ahead and ask. Can the way we breathe really make that much of a difference? I suggest that you try it now. Take a nice long deep belly breath, hold it in for a few seconds and then let it out slowly. How does that feel? Take a few in a row and notice the minor shifts in your physical, mental, and emotional state.

When you take a deep breath, oxygen is allowed to enter your lungs and be exposed to approximately one quart of your blood; within seconds this oxygenation process is delivered to every cell in the body.

You've probably heard of the popularity of Oxygen Bars. It's for this very reason. Improved oxygenation is credited with significant health improvements. Perhaps you've heard the saying, "Disease cannot exist in an oxygenated body." This has been proven by many scientific studies and that is why this is our #1 fundamental of health.

When oxygen is deprived from your cells (especially brain cells), this creates serious consequences very rapidly. The brain can withstand between three to six minutes without oxygen before brain damage occurs. If the brain goes without oxygen for a longer period of time, serious and potentially irreversible damage takes place. After ten minutes, severe neurological damage has generally occurred. Very few people regain any cognitive function after the brain has gone 15 or more minutes without oxygen. Most will not survive beyond this point.

When taking short and shallow breaths, there are cumulative consequences to this low level depletion of oxygen. Over years and decades, this type of breathing impacts the brain and nervous system (the controller of all bodily functions) affecting every cell in our bodies. In the end, shallow breathing creates significant stress to the body, and leads to "fight or flight" nervous system dominance. This puts

continuous pressure on your adrenal function –
a topic that's thoroughly covered in this book.

Action Step:

To increase cellular oxygenation, take three to
five deep belly breaths every waking hour of
your day. Set the timer on your smart phone to
go off hourly or add a reminder using your
favorite timer and BREATHE DEEP.

Here's a sample of a deep belly breathing
exercise:

- Inhale through your nose for
  approximately a count of eight while
  extending your stomach first then the
  chest. Take in as much air as you possible
  can into your lungs.

- Hold that breath for approximately a
  count of four.
- Now exhale this breath through your
  mouth for approximately a count of seven
  while contracting your stomach muscles

to push every bit of breath out. This sets yourself up for the next deep belly breath.

Important Tip:

Committing to this action step supplies your cells with much-needed oxygen. But, there's more good news. One magnificent benefit is that you cannot experience stress at the same time that you take a deep belly breath.

That's pretty remarkable, isn't it.

Also, the more you put this exercise into practice, the more automatic it will become. You are teaching your body a new, healthy pattern of breathing and like any habit, it will eventually become second nature.

Chapter Two

The Water You Drink

This chapter discusses proper hydration of your body. After all, you're made up of approximately 73% water. And, did you know that you can only survive approximately 3 days without water? People can live 3 weeks without food, but without water, survival is just a matter of days.

This fundamental of health is all about getting an optimal quality and quantity of water in on a daily basis.

Let's start with the amount of water to drink daily. The general recommendation is to drink one quart of water for every fifty pounds of body weight. So if you weigh 150 pounds, your daily water intake goal would be three quarts per day.

This is a general recommendation to be adjusted per individual need. There are other factors to take into consideration. After all, we have different activity levels. Some have jobs that require significant movement. Some exercise with regularity and others are more sedentary.

Start with the general recommendation. Additionally, pay attention to the color of your urine to fine tune your personal hydration needs. If your urine is a bright yellow or orange, you need to drink more water. If your urine appears to be clear or colorless, you may be over-hydrated and you may be depleting your electrolyte minerals, which can lead to health challenges.

Ideally look for a very pale yellow color to your urine. This will indicate that you're most likely hydrated properly. As an added note, taking B vitamins could also cause bright colored urine even if you are properly hydrated.

Quantity is not everything though, the quality of your water matters as well. There's a lot of conflicting information on this topic -- even disagreement among health authorities.

Many experts, including myself, believe that in a perfect world, we all would drink natural, unadulterated, spring water. This would be fresh, clean, pure water that's running down a stream accumulating healthy minerals and nutrients. Unfortunately this is difficult to find in the world we live in.

Spring Water

Spring water, as mentioned above, is my preference to recommend. Spring water has been filtered by the earth in ways we do not completely understand. Nature's inexplicable methods are far superior to any man-made means of purifying water. Another advantage is that it contains a wide variety of trace minerals that the human body desperately needs. Ideally, drink only spring water from remote places on earth. As mentioned earlier, this is not always easy to find, but preferred if you find a quality source.

If you cannot confirm a quality source, it may be best to refer to water choices below.

Artesian Water

Artesian water is spring water that comes from a natural underground source. It comes from a well that taps into an underground layer of rock or sand in which the water level rises above the top of the rock. The water is then extracted and bottled.

Reverse Osmosis Water (RO)

This method involves passing water at high pressure through a plastic membrane with tiny holes in it. This is a common filtration method for many bottled water companies as it produces very pure water. There is one caveat here; reverse osmosis takes away the impurities but also the mineral content. If you are using reverse osmosis be sure to add minerals back to this water before drinking it. This can be accomplished by adding liquid mineral drops, Himalayan salt or even a vegetable such as a stalk of celery or fennel. The added bonus of adding a vegetable is often a fresh, delightful, and invigorating flavor.

Alkaline Water

Alkaline water has been ionized to increase its pH to between 8 and 10. Some say alkaline water is beneficial because of its alkalinity (High pH-balance) and ORP (Oxidation Reduction Potential) that makes it an antioxidant. My concern here is that the PH of your blood is approximately 7.2 and when you take something in below or above this PH level, your body will have to convert it back to the pH of 7.2 to be properly utilized. If you are using an alkaline filtration system, I suggest setting this as close to the PH of your blood as you can.

While I am not what you would consider a major supporter of alkaline water, this is still a much better option than most bottled water on the market. And, it's definitely superior to the compromised, and even toxic, water that comes out of your tap.

Tap Water

Tap water contains heavy metals, fluoride, chlorine, medicines like antibiotics and antidepressants and hundreds of chemicals. Many of these "ingredients" in your water are neither measured nor regulated. Fluoride has been noted to cause many side effects such as weakened bones and increased susceptibility to develop osteoporosis and cancer. Yet, it's added to almost every municipal water supply in the country! If tap water is your only viable option I would recommend, at a minimal level, adding a carbon filtration system to improve the quality of your tap water.

Distilled Water

Distilled water has gone through a rigorous filtration process to strip it not only of contaminants, but all natural minerals, leaving this even more "mineral dead" than reverse osmosis water. When water is distilled, by boiling it and condensing it, all solid matter is extracted-except chemicals that were in the water. Most industrial distillers have methods to capture these substances to prevent them from remaining in the water. Because of the mineral void, distilled water grabs and eliminates minerals from the body, a process called chelation. If you are using this form of water, mineral replacement is a must. *I do not recommend drinking this water.*

Mineral Water

Mineral water is extracted from an underground spring and contains natural salts and sulfur compounds. It comes in two forms, still or effervescent. It contains natural mineral as opposed to mineralized water, which are added later. This is another quality source of water for consumption. Be sure that this is naturally carbonated though. If the bottle says carbonation is added, this is not your best option.

Sparkling Mineral Water

My wife calls this, "fizzy water." But, what makes it fizzy? This type of water contains the same amount of carbon dioxide that it had when it emerged from its source. Sparkling bottled waters may be labeled as sparkling drinking water, sparkling mineral water, sparkling or spring water. If choosing this type of water, confirm that it's naturally sparkling, without or very little carbonation added.

Well Water

As you can imagine, well water contamination levels vary widely based on its location. This is especially the case if you live near industrial or agricultural areas. Even if your location appears to be optimal, wells can easily become contaminated with minerals such as iron and manganese. State regulatory testing often fails to test for all detrimental contaminates. If you have a well, have it thoroughly tested before using it for drinking purposes.

Bottled Water

The use of bottled water pollutes the environment and is often nothing more than tap water, not to mention Xenoestrogens that leach into the water from the cheap plastic.

When you must use bottled water, choose brands with high quality scores on EWG's (Environmental Working Group a non-profit organization) Bottled Water Scorecard A-F. Choose water that has been scored closer to A. Typically the thicker plastic bottles are better than the thinner plastic.

If you do use bottled water, please recycle.

Chapter Three

The Food You Eat

"Let food be thy medicine and medicine be thy food."

Hippocrates

You've heard the statement, "you are what you eat," haven't you? I'm going to take it one step further. We live in a time when the majority of people walking have gut challenges whether they're aware of it or not. Gut challenges create a whole cascade of problems with one major challenge today. Many of us are experiencing improper breakdown and utilization of the nutrients from the foods we eat.

Did you know that you can make extremely healthy nutritional choices, yet actually be malnourished? I like to say, **we are NOT what we eat, we are what we absorb and assimilate.** Meaning we are the foods we can actually break down and turn into energy.

There are some quick and simple ways you can analyze your own body to determine the health of your gut. Traditional Chinese Medicine (TCM) has mastered this form of "body communication" and has used it as a diagnostic tool for over 2500 years.

Let me show you what I mean.

Here are some examples of how Traditional Chinese medicine can help you.

Action Step:

Look in the mirror at your tongue. If you notice a vertical crack in the mid portion of the top of your tongue as pictured on the next page, this represents potential chronic challenges with your stomach and/or small intestines.

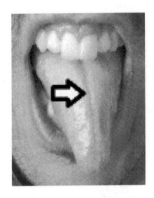

Mid Tongue Crack

Look at your fingernails. Do you have any vertical ridges? This may signify low stomach acid which leads to improper breakdown of your protein, minerals and B vitamins.

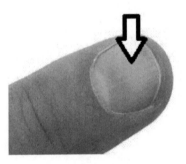

Vertical Ridges

Your body reveals many other signs that can indicate internal issues.

- Do you have horizontal dips in the surface of your fingernail(s)? This is an indication of digestive challenges.

- Have you ever noticed floating stool (bowel movement) in the toilet? This can indicate a compromised ability to breakdown fats in your diet.

- Diarrhea may be a sign of pathogens (bacteria, virus, parasites, etc.) leaky gut, or other digestive issues.

- Constipation indicates potential challenges with your gut/brain connection.

- Acid reflux, also known as GERD, and becoming bloated after meals are two other signs of a decreased ability to absorb and assimilate your food properly. Most often this is caused by low stomach acid due to stress or infection.

If you observe any of these examples, that's good news. You now have the opportunity to do something about it.

When I was healing my gut, I sought the advice and guidance of a well-educated health professional. Together, we took the following steps to help me heal. I highly recommend you start here as well.

- If you notice your stool floating, you may need some liver and/or gall bladder support for improved breakdown of fat.

- Introduce beneficial bacteria (the good bacteria) into your diet through raw fermented vegetables such as kimchi or raw cultured dairy or goat's milk (raw yogurt or kefir). You can also accomplish this by simply taking a Pre/Probiotic capsule that has at least seven strains of the good bacteria, including a food source for the good bacteria. I specially formulated the Depke Wellness Prebiotic/Probiotic Formula because I could not find one that met my standards.

- Take a digestive enzyme just before each meal you consume that includes cooked foods. Raw foods contain natural enzymes needed for proper breakdown of your foods. When food is cooked, the naturally occurring enzymes are damaged and/or destroyed. Adding a digestive enzyme increases the breakdown and absorption of the foods you eat. Choosing one that's appropriate for your particular diet, can be overwhelming. That's what prompted me to formulate one that breaks down flesh proteins including beef, chicken, fish and eggs, fats, carbohydrates, cruciferous vegetables and beans. This specialized, comprehensive formulation is called the

Depke Wellness Prime Enzyme Support.

- If you're dealing with chronic constipation, I recommend reaching out to a qualified natural health practitioner and/or a colon hydro-therapist. Or, you may wish to begin a regimen of home enemas. Colon motility is regulated by the brain and often is tied into a deeper brain issue which we discuss later in this book.

- If you're experiencing painful acid reflux or GERD, this is most often tied into low stomach acid which leads to the inability to properly breakdown proteins in your stomach. You can often stimulate stomach acid production by introducing bitters, cayenne pepper or apple cider vinegar into your diet. You can also attain this through taking a capsule of the *Depke Wellness Prime Stomach Acid Support.* If you are going to use stomach acid supplementation, be sure to confirm that you do not have ulcers, as this could be irritating. The majority of people who experience bloating or constipation after a meal are most often living with low stomach acid.

- A vital step in your healing process is to test for food sensitivities and this is one of the biggest challenges I see with most clients. I will get deeper into this vitally important topic later in this book.

- If you become bloated and/or gassy after certain meals you may have a different issue in your small intestines than lack of enzymes or stomach acid. This health challenge is called "SIBO" or Small Intestinal Bacteria Overgrowth. If SIBO is the culprit, you will bloat and/or get gassy after consuming sugary foods, breads, starchy vegetables and foods, or fibrous foods. SIBO is a common issue for those with long term chronic or on again/off again constipation. SIBO can be tested in one of two ways. First, I recommend mixing one tablespoon of plantain flour (which can be purchased online or in some health food stores) with 16 ounces of water. Drink this on an empty stomach. Wait 20-30 minutes and if you begin to experience bloating or gas, there is a good chance you have SIBO. At this point I highly recommend the more extensive breath test which is done at home and sent to a laboratory for confirmation. If SIBO is present, there's a very specific diet required to follow, along with a supplement regiment. This can make an enormous (not to mention rapid) impact on your health and can be extremely life changing.

- Gut pathogens such as detrimental bacteria, parasites, protozoa, H-pylori and more also contribute to many health challenges, especially if you have experienced a change in your digestion and elimination after traveling out of the country. But let's not kid ourselves, this can happen just as easily eating out and even eating at home. Pathogens can easily be tested with a stool sample kit from your health care provider. I see this with clients on a regular basis and this too can make a huge impact on your health.

- Lastly, other challenges to consider are related to your liver and brain health. If you've experienced long term weight challenges, fatigue, constipation, diarrhea, bloating and other gut issues, you may wish to take the following steps. A quick way to check is to look under your tongue for dark, bulging, or branching veins as pictured on the next page. Also, check for little red specks (like those pictured on page 45) that look like tiny moles on the torso of your body called cherry angiomas, this would indicate liver challenges that need to be addressed. It's important to understand that your gut and brain are connected. Approximately 90% of your brain output goes straight down the spinal column through what's called the Vagus nerve. It travels into the nervous system tissue of the gastrointestinal (GI) system and surrounding organs and then directly back up. So when there's an issue in the gut, there's an issue in the brain and vise-versa.

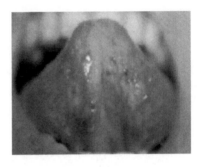

Bulging Veins

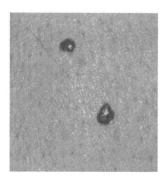

Cherry Angiomas

Food Sensitivity

Food sensitivity is one of the biggest challenges for those struggling with weight issues, fatigue, and frustration. Have you ever eaten a meal and within 20 minutes felt drained of energy, or perhaps you became bloated soon after? These are just two of the many signs of food sensitivity. I need to stress that 86% of food sensitivities, including gluten sensitivity are asymptomatic, meaning that the offending foods can cause internal issues without any apparent physical reaction. Eventually, the undiagnosed food sensitivity will rear its ugly head in a seemingly unrelated "symptom" or illness.

Some of the newest research shows the one of the underlying causes of food sensitivity is due to the fact that we do not digest our protein properly and this is whether this is an animal or plant based protein. We discussed this earlier when talking about low stomach acid.

Another reason some of these foods may create problems for you is that they include Genetically Modified Organisms (GMO), which have been "engineered" in ways foreign to nature. Also, if they are conventionally grown, they may be sprayed with herbicides, pesticides, other chemicals and are highly processed.

Whenever possible, I recommend eating organic, seasonal and locally grown fruit and vegetables, organic, grass-fed, free-range and wild caught meats, poultry, fish, and eggs. If you are dining out make healthy food choices and eat at restaurants that use local organic produce and high quality meat, foul, fish and seafood when possible.

The following is a list of foods I have found with the highest sensitivity for the health-challenged clients I see most frequently.

Take a look and see how many of these foods you eat on a regular basis?

Coffee	Corn	Soy	Cow's Milk
Oats	Yeast	Casein	Whey Protein
Sesame	Buckwheat	Sorghum	Millet
Chocolate	Hemp	Amaranth	Quinoa
Egg	Polish Wheat	Rice	Potato
Wheat	Rye	Barley	Spelt

Imagine if you had one or two of these food sensitivities unbeknownst to you and ate them frequently. If you're eating them and are sensitive to these foods, you are unintentionally creating inflammation and other internal issues that are contributing to your health challenges. Once you know what specific food sensitivities you have, you can eliminate them and begin to reverse the damage they've caused.

Trust me when I say this, food sensitivity will make you fat, fatigued and frustrated!

What's the big deal about food sensitivity anyway?

Food sensitivity creates inflammation in the body which triggers challenges with digestion, physical energy, hormone imbalance, brain, and immune function. Additionally, autoimmune challenges such as Hashimoto's, endometriosis, arthritis, ulcerative colitis and others may result.

There are four food sensitivity tests that I have found to be very accurate and invaluable with helping people lose weight, decrease inflammation, improve gut and brain health, decrease stress, and improve sleep. They are:

- Cyrex Labs Array #3 Wheat/Gluten Reactivity test
- Cyrex Labs Array #4 Gluten Associated Cross Reactive Food Sensitivity test
- ImmunoLabs Bloodprint154
- Array #10 from Cyrex for more extensive testing

These are not "over the counter" tests and you will need to work with a holistic practitioner to have them ordered for you.

One man's food is another man's poison.

2600 years ago a very wise man by the name of Hippocrates said, "One man's food, is another man's poison." This is just as true today as it was then. You are unique. You have a natural, personalized, customized bio-chemical individuality that makes you different from everybody else on the planet.

What this means is that you respond to food very differently than your friends and the same diet might have drastically different results for the two of you. This is why the latest fad diets don't work for everyone.

You are unique based on your genetic makeup, the climate you live in, your varied stress levels, your functional health challenges, your food sensitivities and many other unique details all of which will impact your nutritional needs.

So which diet is best for you?

- Atkins
- Ornish
- South Beach
- Paleo
- High Protein
- High Carb/Low Carb
- Vegetarian
- Vegan

You must know what I mean, right? Think about all of the different diets you have tried, that failed you! You didn't fail, the diet failed you.

And here's why.

From a genetic factor it's important to understand that it takes our bodies many generations to create a shift in nutritional needs. Many cultures have thrived with optimal health based on the foods that were locally and seasonally available to them, not foods that have been packaged and shipped half way around the world as in today's culture.

Did you know that traditional Eskimos thrived in an extremely challenging climate with their main dietary intake being only fat and protein? They experienced virtually no heart disease, no high blood pressure and no cancer.

The Aborigines consumed much more vegetation, insects, kangaroo and wallaby meat, yet had the strength and fitness of Olympic athletes.

The Swiss consumed large amounts of high fat cheese, raw milk, small amounts of protein, whole rye and some wine yet survived very well even through glacier winters.

The African Masai consumed raw milk, meat and blood from cattle yet enjoyed superb mental and physical development.

I'm not necessarily recommending these particular diets. What I am recommending is moving closer to your true genetic, bio-individual nutritional needs. I have seen amazing things happen when people like you make this change.

As a bonus for you, we offer this assessment referred to as your Nutritional ID. If you visit DepkeWellness.com and click on the word Specialties in the upper heading, you will find this assessment under Nutritional ID.

Discover your Nutritional ID today.

I've seen stubborn excess weight drop off easily and effortlessly. I've witnessed optimized energy levels, decreased internal stress levels, improved sleep, balanced hormones, transformed digestion, and so much more.

I'd love to see this happen for you too!

It's all about moderation, or is it?

I'd like to address a common misconception that eating "everything in moderation" is the nutritional ideal we should strive to achieve. Imagine yourself living many years ago, significantly north of the equator and before the industrial revolution. You would never have tasted a grapefruit, orange, pineapple, kiwi or other produce grown in areas far from you. We're now told to consume these foods on a regular basis -- and year round.

While the foods listed above would have been foreign to you, you'd be familiar with fruit such as apples, pears, and berries. You would have enjoyed these fruits only when in season, with only a limited time for consumption.

The same would be true if you lived near the equator. You would have thrived on tropical fruit, vegetation, low fat flesh proteins, warm water fish and seafood. If someone then put you on a high fat, high protein diet, this could prove disastrous.

Another common misconception, in my opinion, is the belief that it's beneficial to eat many small meals per day. I can share that from my years of nutritional research and work with thousands of individual clients who want to lose weight, increase energy, combat disease and truly be healthy, this simply is not true. I've witnessed this over and over. When you consume meals that are right for your nutritional needs, then you will feel completely satiated, and enjoy high core energy physically, mentally, and emotionally. All of these benefits are yours, with no more than three balanced meals per day.

Fat Burning Mode

Fat burning mode is based on the duration of time between meals. Once you eat a meal, your body will use the nutrients from that food to produce energy for the next 3 hours. After 3 hours you will begin burning fat. This fat provides higher levels of energy compared to burning carbohydrates from a meal which is key to losing weight and having optimal health.

We all want to lose fat and enjoy increased energy, don't we?

A big mistake is eating too often. Anytime 25 calories or more are eaten the body shifts from fat burning mode into food burning mode.

So think about this the next time you reach for a few almonds between meals (which contain 28 calories). All of your energy for the next 3 hours will be fueled by these few almonds which typically will have you reaching for another snack in no time.

As your health and nutrition improve, waiting 4 to 6 hours between meals will occur naturally.

For a small percentage, snacking between meals is a genetic need. Others with health challenges may have a function need to snack between meals. If you are this person, make sure you keep your snack 25 calories or less.

Here are some under 25 calorie snack ideas

- Super green drink powder mixed with water and be sure to confirm it is 25 calories or less (We recommend the *Depke Wellness Prime Organic Greens & Reds*)
- 1 medium stalk of celery is only 6 calories
- 25 blueberries
- 1 small to medium size carrot
- 5 medium strawberries

Follow these guidelines and enjoy burning fat and improved energy.

Action Steps:

- As mentioned earlier, you'll be happy to know that I created a simple way to assess your nutritional individuality. I've done the work for you. It's a proven method that teaches you a way to tap into your own body's wisdom while fine tuning your nutritional needs. Upon completion of this easy to do assessment, you'll know what type of foods your body needs right now and how much. I invite you to visit www.DepkeWellness.com and take my free, quick Nutritional ID assessment. You will find this listed under the Specialties section at the very top left of the website.

- Once you've discovered your Nutritional ID, you now have a starting point. You can begin to eat the foods that are recommended, allowing a minimum of four to five hours between meals. If you feel you're not able to go this long between meals, this is an indication of deeper health issues that will need to be addressed first. If you are able to go 4, 5, even 6 hours between meals, wonderful. You're on your way to efficiently burning fat and allowing your body to rebuild and repair, thereby creating optimal levels of health for you.

Chapter Four

Your Sleep

Imagine how delighted you will feel when you wake up from the deepest, most restful sleep you have ever experienced. You'll feel happy, energized and excited for the new day! Sounds amazing, doesn't it.

The quality of your sleep is vital to your health, happiness and daily energy levels. This also has a direct link to weight gain and fatigue. During the hours of deep sleep your body and immune system completes most of your cellular repair and maintenance. This is absolutely necessary for optimal health and wellbeing.

Simply put, high quality sleep is essential.

You're probably now wondering how you can get some, right. The following factors are related to high quality sleep and your success with achieving this deep healing state.

- The time you go to sleep
- Your duration of sleep
- The quality of your sleep
- The time you wake up
- How you feel when you get up
- Protein and your sleep
- Hormones and your sleep

Time and Duration of Sleep

As a general rule, we should all strive to achieve approximately eight hours of sleep. Some may need slightly more and others slightly less. Not only do we have personal variances but these often shift seasonally.

We typically require more sleep in the winter months and less sleep in the summer. Ideally, go to bed before or close to 9:30 pm in the winter months and before or close to 10:30 pm in the summer months.

You may be one who goes to bed at what you think is a reasonable hour. And then you toss and turn all night, never achieving deep, restorative sleep. Or, maybe you're a "night person" who stays up late and believes you only need a few hours of sleep to function. My response is always the same, "there's no such thing as a night person." This is simply a learned behavior or a part of deeper functional issues. These functional issues generally involve adrenal (energy) gland function which governs energy levels, hormone function, and/or digestive function. I'll expand upon this later in this chapter.

Sleep is a self-regulated factor that's directly tied into sun exposure and the magnetic variances of the earth. Therefore, becoming a "night person" is a learned behavior. The good news is that as a behavior, it can be "unlearned."

Sleep is essentially important for your adrenal gland function, which is tied into just about every function of your body. This includes regulation of all hormone production, has a significant impact on energy levels, and your overall health and happiness. Poor adrenal function is a key culprit in feeling fat, fatigued and frustrated as well as creating sickness and disease.

The prime time of repair for your adrenal glands is from 9:00 pm to 11:00 pm, so if you're consistently getting to bed after 11:00 pm, you're missing out on this peak opportunity time to rebuild and repair.

The ideal waking time is less complicated than this; simply get up with the sun. The response of your hormone cortisol, is naturally at its highest during the time near the sun rising. This increase in cortisol naturally shifts your body from a sleep state into a waking state for you to start your day. It's also important to gauge *how* you wake up. Remember when you were a child and you woke up early? You probably bounced out of bed! This is the natural balance I want you to rediscover. If you're not waking up this way, then I'd like to help you discover what health challenges are in your way.

Perhaps you're one of those "night people" who goes to bed at 1:00 am and sleeps in the next day. If that's the case, you're not only losing the prime time of repair for the glands responsible for generating energy, but you're also missing the spike in cortisol that helps you wake naturally.

Very often, those who claim to be "night people" share with me that they get so much done at night time. But in the long run, this sleep pattern consistently creates deeper, functional challenges for your body. Shifting to an earlier bed time and wake time allows more to be accomplish during the day with peak focus compared to a late night "get it done" binge with impaired faculties.

I've seen this fact repeatedly. You are much better off- from every perspective - going to bed earlier and waking with the sunrise.

This is so important!

Perhaps you're someone who works 2nd or 3rd shifts? If possible I recommend switching to working during the day. If that's not possible you will want to create new habits & behaviors that get you into a relaxed state as soon as you arrive at home. A warm bath or relaxing music can prove helpful as well as drinking chamomile tea.

Action Steps:

- Dim the lights in the house after sunset, or at the latest 9 pm.

- Discontinue watching any TV, phone, tablet, or computer use at least 60 minutes prior to bedtime.

- Get ready for bed around 9:00 or 9:30 every evening, perhaps a bit later in the summer months. Create a nighttime routine of brushing teeth, washing face, getting into your comfy clothes or pajamas, etc.

- Listen to relaxing music, meditate, pray, practice deep breathing, light yoga or stretching, take a hot bath, and/or light reading before bed will help you naturally wind down from your day.

- If you're a "night person" implement these action steps but begin one hour earlier than you currently go to bed for the first few days or week. Then two hours earlier than you originally went to bed. Continue this process until you are regulated back to an ideal sleep pattern.

Now that you're going to bed earlier you're ready for the next step. Let's improve the quality of your sleep! The goal is to sleep completely through the night, naturally flowing through all of levels of sleep without waking. If you wake during the night, decreasing the number of times you wake and increasing your ability to easily and effortlessly fall back asleep quickly is essential. Waking often and having trouble

65

falling back to sleep is another sign of deeper issues that I'll soon address.

Why do some have poor quality sleep?

There are many factors that can contribute to poor quality of sleep. These include but aren't limited to imbalances in the adrenal glands, digestive system, liver, lungs, and colon.

While there may be many ways to address sleep issues, I've found that focusing on adrenal and digestive challenges is the fastest method to achieve this success. Balancing these two systems creates a beautiful cascading effect on sleep and other parts of the body.

This improves health faster and synergistically.

Let's begin with a review of hormone rhythms, specifically the relationship between cortisol (your stress hormone) and melatonin (your sleep hormone). We'll discuss how they play a role in sleep quality.

First, let me explain that the stress hormones and sleep hormones should spike at the exact opposite ends of the time line. If we look at a 24 hour cycle, your stress hormone should ideally be at its highest near 6:00 am, at their lowest near midnight, and then back to its highest again near 6:00 am the next morning. Your sleep hormone should be the exact opposite. Its low point of the day should be near 6:00 am, its highest point near midnight and then back to its low point again near 6:00 am. Because these hormones, cortisol and melatonin, are typically opposites, it's important to watch your nighttime cortisol levels. If your nighttime cortisol, stress hormone, is too high, this creates a lower sleep response. In the end, this creates challenges in falling asleep, staying asleep, and/or causing you to feel tired in the morning.

A simple adrenal saliva test helps me to analyze the stress and sleep hormone levels of my clients. I commonly find lower than optimal sleep hormone levels at night. If melatonin is low, there are two primary reasons. The first being elevated cortisol at night due to stress patterns and secondly, poor or compromised digestion.

At first glance, it may seem that a melatonin supplement is needed but this typically is not the case. What's needed is to discover why your body is not producing the sleep hormone it needs to release at night. This hormone assists with your sleep cycle and creates balance.

Melatonin/Cortisol Rhythm

Midnight

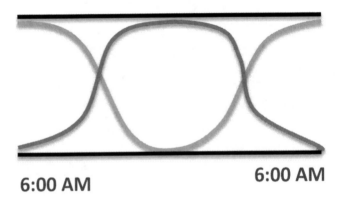

6:00 AM　　　　**6:00 AM**

When your melatonin/cortisol rhythm is in healthy function, your stress hormone (cortisol) is very high in the morning and very low at midnight. The melatonin (sleep hormone) would be very low in the morning and very high at midnight. When these two hormones are in proper rhythm they will be exact opposites throughout the day, and leave you sleeping well. If your cortisol is too high in the evening due to some form of chronic stress, this will push your melatonin to a lower level, created sleep issues on two different levels. Fist the lack of melatonin to initiate a proper sleep cycle and second, your cortisol is stimulated and keeping you awake and alert.

Look at the link between melatonin, your sleep hormone levels and protein.

This breakdown on the next page will illustrate how the combination of protein consumption with digestive function ties into your melatonin production.

Here's what's necessary for proper conversion of protein into melatonin, your sleep hormone:

1. Protein consumption (at least once every 24 hour period)
2. Proper digestion and breakdown of protein
3. Breakdown of protein to amino acids
4. Protein breaks down into L-tryptophan
5. L-tryptophan breaks down into 5-HTP
6. 5-HTP breaks down into Serotonin
7. Serotonin breaks down into Melatonin

To help increase the quality of your sleep, be sure you're eating a quality source of meat or egg protein at least every 24 hours. If you're consuming a vegetarian or vegan diet, you'll need to carefully combine your plant proteins in order to take in proper essential amino acids for this conversion to take place. If you are vegan, it's also vital to supplement with vitamin B12.

Once you're consuming a small amount of protein at least every 24 hours, it's important to optimize your digestive function. Here's a reminder of my favorite mantra, you're not what you eat but what you absorb and assimilate.

I often see clients who eat very well, yet they're still malnourished.

This has a significant impact on their melatonin production and sleep patterns. With proper digestion, protein breakdown into essential amino acids (referring to the amino acids you must get from food). These amino acids are the building blocks of life as we know it. They also play a major role in brain function and production of neurotransmitters which are brain chemicals that communicate information throughout the brain, the gut, and the rest of the body.

One of these amino acids is L-tryptophan. You probably relate this to the element in turkey that makes us sleepy after Thanksgiving dinner. Most of your L-tryptophan is used in the production of B vitamins and other functions in your body. But a small percentage is used as a part of this conversion from protein eventually into melatonin. This small percentage converts to the naturally occurring amino acid 5-HTP, which then converts to the neurotransmitter serotonin. Serotonin itself is a chemical neurotransmitter that helps regulate mood, behavior, anxiety, appetite, and pain sensation. It also converts into melatonin.

You can see from this diagram below, the flow from protein consumption to melatonin, your sleep hormone, has a few stops along the way.

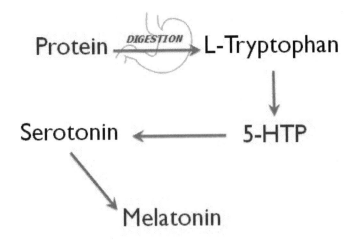

There are so many other essential components for your body to complete throughout this entire process. It should now be clear how important it is to take care of this at the core with proper protein uptake and healthy digestion.

For more tips, please refer back to the section on improving your digestion in *The Food You Eat Section* beginning on page 42 of this book. You can begin to implement some of the recommendations referenced there to optimize your digestion and improve the quality of your sleep.

Serotonin -- Your "Happy Hormone" and Sleep

Proper serotonin production in the body plays an important role in sleep. Scientists have found that serotonin directly promotes wakefulness and also promotes the formation of sleep-promoting brain factors.

This allows us to be alert, awake, and sleepy all at proper times.

Estrogen hormones play a direct role with serotonin levels. For example, if estrogen levels are high, symptoms of serotonin excess are created. If estrogen is low, this can cause symptoms of low serotonin activity. Because of the estrogen/serotonin connection, taking supplements to support serotonin may not achieve the results you're looking for. This is particularly true if you're estrogen deficient. How would you know? A comprehensive adrenal panel (saliva test) can provide this answer.

You'll find detailed information about this subject in the *Bonus Section* starting on page 164 of this book.

Tryptophan and 5-HTP

Both 5-HTP and tryptophan have been shown to assist in increasing serotonin levels. They can help address the symptoms caused by low serotonin. Both of these substances are precursors to serotonin production and I often suggest the use of both to assist serotonin production.

Iron and Serotonin

The production of your happy hormone (serotonin) depends on adequate levels of iron. Therefore, iron deficiency is an important factor to consider when addressing low serotonin. This is common for those who follow a vegan or vegetarian diet and for those with low stomach acid production. One of the most common challenges that would lead to low stomach acid production is the presence of an H-pylori infection.

Nutritional Deficiencies

There are many nutrients that are essential to synthesize your happy hormones in your body. Adding to the list mentioned above, we can also add vitamin B6, niacin, vitamin B12, folate, and magnesium.

Improving Your Success

If you are experiencing happy hormone deficiencies and supplements alone are not creating a positive shift, then I'd recommend addressing some of the typical areas that could potentially sabotage your success. This includes improving general brain health; implementing ways to decrease chronic stress, correct blood sugar imbalances, and decrease alcohol consumption. Brain health, the stress response and blood sugar all have an intimate connection with your adrenal function.

What does your liver, lungs, and colon have to do with sleep?

Your sleep patterns and sleep dysregulation can be connected to challenges with your liver, lungs, and/or colon function. In Traditional Chinese Medicine the energetic time of the liver is between 1:00 am to 3:00 am, the time of the lungs is between 3:00 am to 5:00 am and the time of the colon is from 5:00 am to 7:00 am. So, if you're waking with consistency during any of these time frames, this could be a sign of deeper functional issues with the corresponding organ.

Recommendations for healing the liver and colon are listed in the next section of this book titled *Movement* and recommendations for the lungs are listed in *the Air You Breath* section pages 20-24.

Further Action Steps to Improve Your Sleep:

- Don't drink water or other beverages past 8:00 pm. If proper sleep eludes you, perhaps a small cup of chamomile or sleepy time tea near 8:00 pm will help you relax. Do you want to mention alcohol before bed? For many, it's a stimulant, not a relaxant.

- A few hours before bed take the time to connect positively with your loved one(s). Bedtime isn't the time to hash out challenges or conflicts. It's a time to simply connect, share about each other's day, and talk about goals and dreams.

- Bedtime is also a good time to jot down things you wish to remember or add to your "to do" list. By writing down items that need to be done the next day or in the future, you're taking concerns off your mind. This helps to quiet the mind and provide a more relaxed state that that may lead to deeper sleep.

- Be sure your sleeping area is completely dark and free from ambient light (windows, electronics, etc.). Sleeping in a darkened room naturally increases your happy hormone. Close your blinds or shut your drapes completely. If you have thin blinds or drapes, I'd even go as far as recommend purchasing room darkening shades (or black out shades) to block out the light entirely.

- Any light that you may use on your nightstand lamp, be sure to use a light bulb with a red tint. The typically light bulb will put out a blue light which will inhibit melatonin while the red light will enhance melatonin. This is also why using electronics before bed, which tend to put off a blue light, are so detrimental to sleep.

- Cover any lit items in your bedroom, such as a LED clock, the light on the front of your cable receiver, etc.

- Listen to a hypnotic or relaxation CD or recording before bedtime.

- I only recommend supplement sleep aids in extreme circumstances. Typically, if you follow the tips listed above, address adrenal function, and improve your digestion, then proper sleep patterns will no longer be a problem.

Have fun implementing these new action steps. You'll enjoy improved sleep patterns, and reap the deep level benefits that sleep plays in your health and wellness goals.

Chapter Five

Movement

"If we could give every individual the right amount of nourishment and exercise, not too little and not too much, we would have found the safest way to health."

Hippocrates

What comes to mind when you think of the word movement?

"Movement" is a very broad term that can take on many meanings. We are going to discuss three very important and specific types of movements; the types that are best for losing weight and improving energy.

- Movement of the Body
- Movement of the Spine
- Movement of the Colon

Movement of the Body

What if you could stop your intense workouts and lose weight? How about never visit a gym, yet still attaining all of your exercise goals?

Sounds great, right?

To start, I ask you to set aside all of the current knowledge you have on the subject of exercise. I'd like you to be free from preconceived ideas as I share insights and new understandings regarding the type of movement/exercise that's best for losing weight, increasing energy, and creating a healthy body from the inside out

We live in a culture that values "more is better." Applying this "more" philosophy to most areas of life can could prove detrimental to our overall health and happiness.

For example, let's apply it to exercise. Extreme activities such as running marathons and competing in triathlons fatigue and exhaust the body in many ways. When these intense extreme athletes come to me for help, they soon recognize the impact that extreme exercise has on their overall health. But for many, it's a passion they're not willing to give up.

If you find yourself in this category of athletics it's essential to find a knowledgeable health practitioner who can create a custom fitness program that includes significant nutritional and supplemental support during training and competitions. Additionally, an extensive rebuilding protocol needs to be implemented during the off season. This most often includes helping your body rebuild your stressed out adrenal system.

Is high intensity exercise helping or hindering you?

Because you're a person who cares about your health, it's important to understand that intense aerobic training has the potential to create health challenges or worsen your current issues. Pushing your heart rate to its maximum level and maintaining this heightened state of exertion for extended periods of time, stalls the healing process and destroys the body's ability to repair and rebuild.

While these forms of exercise below may be fine for the person in optimal health and proper hormone (adrenal) balance, those that are feeling fat, fatigued and frustrated, these are more likely hindering, rather than helping you.

Action Step:

Eliminate the following methods of exercise.

- Aerobic classes
- Spin classes
- High intensity yoga
- Running
- Biking with sustained intensity
- Circuit training without rest between sets

Almost any form of intense exercise that doesn't allow the heart rate to normalize at least periodically, fits into this category.

So many people are suffering through these intense workouts, feeling exhausted and depleted and not getting the results that they are looking for. Isn't the thought of stopping this exciting to you?

Or maybe you're at the opposite end of the spectrum.

Perhaps you feel guilty because you "know" you should be working out to the point of utter exhaustion, yet you can't push yourself that hard, or maybe you haven't even started.

Congratulations!

Take a deep breath and release any guilt or regret you may have over your fitness intentions. I'm going to share with you the type of movement that'll provide the exact results you desire.

What type of exercise is best?

The body is designed to move.

Movement is one of the fundamentals of health that helps you create the body of your dreams. You can create a body that slips into your skinny jeans easily and effortlessly and ensures that you fully engaged in life, feeling energetic and happy with the new you!

The key is to figure out the best type of exercise to suit your current needs.

While some people have a genetic makeup that enables them to tolerate aerobic training, for the rest of us, finding a less intense, or moderate, form of movement is ideal. This is especially true if you're challenged in any way with your health. Moderate exercise includes anaerobic training that raises the heart rate and allows it to come back down to normal levels rather quickly.

Examples of anaerobic training include:

- All types of sprints (running, biking, etc.) with sprints in short bursts of 30 seconds followed by one to two minutes of casual movement
- Jumping rope with a high intensity for 30 seconds followed by walking in place for two minutes
- Hill climbing intensely for 30 seconds with casual movement for two minutes after
- Walking with an exaggerated arm swing
- Heavy weight-lifting with low reps and rest in-between sets
- Burst training

Most of these are examples of "burst training." The definition of burst training is any movement such as running, biking, pushups, crunches, squats, jumping jacks, or rebounding (jumping on a mini trampoline) at an intense capacity for only 30 seconds, followed by two minutes of slow casual movement. An example of this could be completing 30 seconds of vigorous jumping jacks (doing them as fast as humanly possible) followed by two minutes of walking in place.

NOTE: Rebounding (a non-impact activity) is the desired recommendation for those with mobility issues and/or joint pain concerns.

I recommend no more than 20 minutes per burst training session (eight – 30 second bursts followed by eight - two minute periods of casual movement) and no more than three burst training sessions per week.

If you're new to burst training, you may find that you need to start with five or ten minutes max and work your way up.

I do want to mention that if you are not in condition to exercise in this manner, do not jump directly into burst training. I recommend getting permission from your doctor to confirm your fitness level and determine if you're in adequate shape to engage in this activity.

The body not only needs fitness activities on a daily basis, it also thrives from daily stretching and restorative movements. I highly recommend doing a variety of the following movements and changing them up weekly.

You'll discover joy in the art of fitness.

As your body begins to move, your breathing deepens, your stress levels decrease, your sleep improves, and deep healing begins.

- Casual morning, lunchtime, or evening walk
- Casual 20-30 minute bike ride
- Stretching, gentle movements, and/or walking in a pool
- Gentle/therapeutic/restorative yoga
- Gentle and slow stretching in the morning upon waking and before bed
- Slow body weight movements (sometimes as simple as getting up and down from a chair ten times in a row every other day)
- Using the stairs instead of the elevator

- Parking in a parking spot at the mall/grocery store that's furthest away from the entrance

As you begin implementing these new restorative movements into your life, you'll discover they're more fun than you imagined. Try a variety of different activities until you find one or two that you thoroughly enjoy. You may wish to even mix them up seasonally. You may find you prefer different movements in the summer vs. the winter.

Variety is good.

Accountability

When committing to a new habit, follow through is often much easier when we have someone besides ourselves to hold us accountable. I recommend finding an accountability partner to commit to an exercise routine with you. You may wish to commit to walking together three times a week, take a restorative yoga class, join a gym, or hire a personal trainer together. Be sure to keep the exercise on an anaerobic level to enhance your health and improve the function of your entire body.

Spinal Movement

I'm not a Chiropractic doctor but I support quality Chiropractic care. Because this isn't my expertise, I've asked a friend and colleague to write this section of the book. I'd like to introduce you to Dr. William Janeshak, founder and CEO of Yorba Linda Family Chiropractic in Southern California. He's truly an expert in the dynamic field of spinal movement.

Why Spinal Movement and Spinal Care?

"Because I said so," and, "I am a doctor," doesn't cut it anymore. In today's world, people are way too smart just to listen to an authority figure and do what they say. Especially when it's a treatment protocol that's been so misunderstood in the past.

As a chiropractor, I work with the nervous system first and foremost. Your nervous system was the first system developed when you were in your mother's belly. The nervous system is referred to as the "Master System" of the entire body because of its regulatory control over all other systems of the body. It sounds pretty important, doesn't it?

Let me explain.

As a Chiropractor I not only have expertise regarding the muscular system and body movement, I'm actually closer to a Neurologist in my training. Chiropractors are "Natural Doctors." We understand that by supporting the body with the basics and removing nerve interference throughout the spine the body has what it needs to heal naturally. We do not prescribe drugs and we do not perform surgeries. We don't manipulate the body's natural chemistry and we do not remove anything that helps the body do its job. A spinal adjustment reduces and relieves interference in the nerve pathways. It increases the powerful communication from the brain through the spinal cord and nervous system to the rest of the body.

The nervous system is so vital that it's the only system of the entire body that's completely encased in bones for protection. The brain is protected by the skull and the spinal cord is sheltered by 24 moveable bones called vertebrae. The spinal cord is connected to the brain via nerves. The nerves let the brain know what happening to the body and the origins of those signals. All of these movements are calculated in the brain so it can determine how to respond.

Here's an example of this complex system in action.

Action Step:

Close your eyes. Reach your hand out in front of your face, make a fist, and extend only your index finger (as if pointing at something). Next, touch the tip of your nose with your extended finger.

Did your finger touch your nose? How did you find your nose with your eyes closed? How did you know exactly where your finger was in relation to your nose?

Your nerves told your brain the location of your finger and nose. Your nerves identified what position your hand was in, how much force you needed to squeeze your fist, the proper angle of your wrist, and the distance your nose was from your face. Your brain makes millions of calculations in seconds just for this one simple action.

Imagine what the brain needs to calculate create and maintain your health!

The magnificent brain also has the same relationship with your organs, tissues, cells, hormones, neurotransmitters, and environment. Most of us are unaware of these processes until something goes wrong.

Waiting for physical pain to appear, is usually what prompts people to seek out care for their spine. Being able to handle pain doesn't mean you're functioning properly. When you're committed to living the best quality of life, be sure you're firing with all cylinders at all times.

Now that you have a basic understanding of the importance of Chiropractic care, how the nervous system is the Master System, and how a properly functioning nervous system is a key to achieving and maintaining your health, you might ask this question. How does my spine get out of alignment? Great question!

Here are three main culprits that trigger misalignment.

1. Physical Stress
2. Chemical Stress
3. Emotional Stress

Physical Stress and Your Spine:

Physical stress occurs from traumatic incidents such as car accidents, sports injuries, or improperly lifting something awkward or heavy. It can also occur from repetitive activities such as using a computer mouse all day or frequently participating in a one-handed sport. These all have a huge impact on both the spine and the nervous system.

Add to this, the subject of poor posture. It's not only unattractive, it pulls the body and the spine out of alignment. This can result in chronic, and sometimes permanent, spinal problems. Sitting or standing in one position for long periods of time also causes the spine to fatigue and fall out of alignment.

While this list is by no means exhaustive, it includes the most common contributors to physical stress.

Chemical Stress and Your Spine

Chemical stress may include food sensitivity or allergies, processed food and genetically modified foods (GMOs), toxins in the environment, and/or chemicals in your body care and cleaning products. It may even include ingredients in your prescribed and over the counter medications.

When we ingest or come in contact with a chemical that the body doesn't recognize, it unleashes a stress response. This response causes the nerves to be hypersensitive and muscles to tighten up, especially around the spine. Consider this, when the body perceives that it's under constant threat, the integrity of the spine can slowly weaken and degenerate. Or, that perceived threat can cause acute spasms throughout the body throwing your spine and nervous system out of balance. This cascades to further body dysfunction.

Despite what you may hear from others, vegetable drinks loaded with GMO's and processed "health" bars are not beneficial to the body. In fact, the food choices you make can have a far greater impact on your health than you imagine.

Emotional Stress and Your Spine

The third way the spine becomes misaligned is related to emotional stress. When you were last stressed out, how did your body react? Did your muscles tighten? Did you get a headache? Did you find it hard to concentrate?

I've known many people who keep themselves fit, and eat very healthy, but are always anxious. They worry about every little thing and are therefore constantly sick.

Learning to take control of your emotions can easily help you to take control of your health. The fact is that your worries, fears, and anxieties only have as much power as you give them. Putting into practice the simple techniques that you'll find outlined in this book is a great way to begin.

Colon Movement

Have you heard of the children's book *Everyone Poops*? Well, at the risk of stating the obvious, it's true. Everyone poops, but the real question is, how often? I know this subject tends to be taboo and may even be pretty gross to talk about. However I can't let this go unsaid. This topic must be addressed for the sake your overall health and wellbeing.

How many bowel movements do you need to have per day to be considered healthy? One? Two? The shock for me is that most people feel that one bowel movement per day is healthy. Even worse, I've heard of doctors telling their patients that they don't even need to have a bowel movement every day. I was mortified when my friend's infant was only pooping every five days or so and the pediatrician said that it was fine. His justification was that "everybody has their own schedule with bowel movements."

How scary!

Hippocrates said over 2000 years ago that all health and disease begins in the gut. The colon is in charge of efficiently moving waste out of the gut, and frankly, if you're not pooping -- you're not healthy.

After reading this section, you'll completely understand the importance of regular bowel movements, how frequently you should have them, and how to have better ones. I've included some helpful and easy steps for improving this area of your life.

It's all About Movement!

Let me first start by sharing this fact -- the food you eat should move completely through your gastrointestinal tract (GI) in 18 hours or less. So, if you're only having one bowel movement in a 24 hour period, you're not evacuating your bowels completely. Movement of foods through the colon is crucial for optimal health. Flesh proteins (meat and fish), will begin to putrefy in the GI tract (creating gas, bloating, flatulence or worse disturbances) if it's not eliminated efficiently and regularly.

Let's do the simple math.

If you have only one bowel movement daily, you'll have a residual of about six meals in your colon at any given time. Have you ever noticed that little tummy pouch near or just below your belly button? This is often a buildup of un-eliminated fecal matter.

Disgusting to think about, isn't it?

Can you imagine how many meals are stored inside your colon if you only experience one bowel movement per day for years? Add to that, the circumstances of constipation from eating a meal that didn't agree with you, or irregular bowel movements due to changes in your work schedule or travel? Skipping regular bowel movements has a cumulative effect on your digestive system. This results in a significant buildup of residue in the colon. The days, weeks, and years of this buildup can actually move fecal matter into the small intestines.

This can lead to so many other challenges such as but not limited to:

- Nutrient malabsorption
- Bloating and distention
- Liver congestion
- Increased toxicity
- Poor mental clarity
- Mood swings
- Headaches
- Poor comprehension
- Gut pathogens
- Weakened immunity
- Decreased energy levels

One factor that's important to understand at this point is the interaction between colon function and your liver.

The liver is your primary organ of detoxification. It processes a significant amount of your toxic load. The liver converts your fat soluble toxins into water soluble toxins and once converted, these toxins can be eliminated from the body in watery fluids such as bile, sweat, saliva and urine.

Bile is excreted from the liver into bile ducts which empty into the small intestines. Waste is then carried away from the liver and eliminated via the feces through the colon. Bile provides an important pathway for toxins get out of your body via your daily bowel movements. If you're not having at least two healthy bowel movements per day, the toxicity your liver is trying to discard through bile is not eliminated. It then begins to recirculate throughout your body.

This is not how your body's system of elimination was designed to function.

Even worse, now when your liver is going through the conversion process, the recirculated toxins are even more toxic than they were in the first place. So, if you're not evacuating your bowels regularly, you're not simply absorbing the same toxic load, you're absorbing an intensified and even more dangerous toxic load.

Everybody wants to decrease toxicity in their body, not increase it.

Here's another extremely significant factor regarding the frequency of bowel movements per day. If you're not enjoying optimal bowels movements, which is a minimum of two per day, your colon has become a storage unit rather than a transport unit. The walls of the colon are permeable. If you're storing waste materials in the colon, the (toxic) contents will begin to leach their way through the colon walls and into the tissue of the body. Eventually, these toxins recirculate back into your blood stream.

And it's not just a matter of toxins. Potentially, hormones that were marked for release through your colon, may also be become trapped in this recirculation process. In essence, a sluggish colon leads to a toxic response and hormone imbalance that affects the whole body.

So what is an optimal bowel movement?

You should have at least two healthy bowel movements per day. Achieve your most substantial bowel movement release in the morning and your second in late afternoon or early evening. If you have multiple bowel movements in the morning, these count as one as this is most likely due to slower motility. When this occurs, the colon doesn't allow a complete release in one sitting.

The basic schedule is this: your afternoon or early evening movement releases your breakfast (from that morning), and the morning movement releases your lunch and dinner from the previous day. This healthy cycle depicts healthy bowel evacuation with no buildup as mentioned earlier.

With a minimum of two bowel movements per day, you're moving your food from the mouth, through your body and out your colon in 18 hours or less. This is essential for ideal health.

Now, if we really want to talk peak perfection here, we'd strive for a bowel movement approximately 30 to 90 minutes after every meal. Does this sound ridiculous to you? Let's think about it. It makes sense. As food goes in, food must come out. If the digestive system is in healthy working order, this timing can be a reality.

A perfect example of this is a healthy, breastfed infant. Within approximately 20 minutes after nursing, this baby poops and continues this cycle after each feeding. This is our bowel movement natural cycle. Unfortunately, most people have not experienced this healthy bowel cycle since infancy, if at all.

Take these simple but powerful steps now to help you achieve regular, optimal bowel movements.

Wake up and drink a 12-18 ounce glass of tepid water.

It's vital to rehydrate the body upon waking. The body's internal repairing and rebuilding process during a good night's sleep is dehydrating to the body. Get into the habit of drinking a large glass of room temperature water first thing every morning. Developing this simple habit can have a significant positive impact on the quantity and quality of your morning bowel movements.

If you do not easily move your colon in the morning or if you depend on your morning coffee to finally relieve your morning bowel movement, this is likely tied in poor adrenal hormone health. Remember earlier when I mentioned that hormone cortisol should be highest when you wake up? Well, this is necessary to initiate a healthy colon release also.

Are you drinking too much during meal time?

Drinking liquids with meals dilutes the stomach acid and enzyme activity needed to properly break down what you eat. To enhance your digestion it is best to stop drinking approximately 30 minutes before meal time and wait to drink again until at least 30 but preferably 60 minutes after your meal.

We already discussed how important proper digestion is to your overall health.

This step is an important one to implement. Get in the habit of drinking your water between meals throughout the day. During or right before the meal, only drink enough water to swallow your digestive aids or any other supplements you may take near meal time. If you must drink during this time, be sure that you drink small amounts, only a few ounces, and drink room temperature or warm liquids.

Drinking a large glass of an ice cold beverage during meal time is a digestive disaster for you.

Chew your food thoroughly

Chew your food in small bites until you think you can't chew it anymore. Then chew it some more. It takes a bit of persistent practice but it's worth it. Chewing thoroughly creates a larger surface area of your food, assisting with breakdown and digestion. Saliva is the first stage of digestion and food begins the breakdown process in the mouth. Chewing also signals the stomach to begin releasing the proper digestive juices, stomach acid and digestive enzymes in preparation for further digestion.

Eat Your Meals in a Relaxed State

Turn off the television and sit at the dining room table during meal time. We live in a fast paced world. We're constantly overstimulated from smartphones, emails, social media, marketing, calls, TV advertisements, devastating news, busy careers, family life, kids, relationships, friendships, athletics, chores, grocery shopping, and more. The list is endless. You may become overwhelmed just thinking about it!

This busy lifestyle in itself creates extreme stress and pressure on the body. This doesn't even account for the issues we aren't addressing, such as the stress of unhealthy relationships, poor communication and repressed emotions.

Stress negatively impacts our nervous system. The parasympathetic portion of your nervous system is the "relaxed" half of your nervous system and it is typically linked to the phrase, "rest and digest." Daily stress in our lives impacts the function of the nervous system as well as the digestive system and the colon specifically. In order to encourage harmony and balance within your nervous system, I suggest taking 3 deep belly breaths before eating each meal. Additionally, take a few more deep breaths during the meal. Deep belly breathing assists in creating a state of relaxation, stimulates the parasympathetic nervous system, and ultimately improves digestion and colon motility.

At least allow meal times to be the one time of the day where you sit, relax and enjoy the moment. Breathe and say, "Ahhhh..."

Take a Quality Prebiotic/Probiotic

Sufficient levels of beneficial (good) bacteria are essential for a healthy gut and for efficient motility of your colon. Quality supplements are likely required for this since most of us don't spend time in the kitchen culturing and fermenting delicious raw foods like yogurt, kefir, and kimchi. It's also unlikely that we make our own beverages like water kefir, coconut water kefir, and ancestral recipe beer and wine full of live beneficial bacteria.

A word of warning, consuming highly processed and mass produced store bought yogurt or kefir is not beneficial. These products don't contain much, if any good bacteria because they are pasteurized (heated) destroying all living bacteria. Sadly, this is the case despite what their ads and labels claim. You may be surprised to learn that it's legal for manufacturers to list the bacteria as "live," because the food did contain living strains prior to pasteurization and after culturing. They simply fail to mention most of the live bacteria is killed during the process.

Of course, *dead* bacteria will serve no purpose at all.

If you prefer capsules, I recommend supplementing with a multiple strain 40 billion+ count of beneficial bacteria each morning upon waking. Take these capsules with your 12-18 ounces of tepid water.

I personally take two *Depke Wellness Prebiotic/Probiotic Formula* to start my day.

Take a Comprehensive Digestive Enzyme

Have you ever had an overcooked chicken breast or piece of steak that just sat in your stomach and felt like an unmovable rock? Or have you experienced a bowel movement that required the use of half a roll of toilet paper afterward? How about feeling uncomfortably bloated after eating a delicious meal that included beans?

These are three signs that you are not properly breaking down proteins and legumes. A digestive aid can help.

Did you know the first third of the stomach is where pre-digestion occurs? The level of pre-digestion that takes place depends on how raw or cooked the food is. All raw foods contain natural occurring enzymes that help the body to break it down easily and efficiently; yet cooking our food destroys these naturally occurring enzymes. Cooking at the temperature of 118 degrees or more will destroy these naturally occurring enzymes and even heating to lower temperatures will degrade the enzyme activity.

If this pre-digestion can't occur, the digestive process further down the pathway is slowed and potentially inefficient.

A high quality digestive enzyme supplement can begin the process of pre-digestion for cooked foods. This is essential if you are eating meat, fish, eggs, healthy fats, beans, cooked vegetables, and grains. Consume an enzyme supplement that contains both quality plant and animal based enzymes helps to break down the cooked foods you consume in an optimal manner.

Please read your product labels. If you're using an enzyme supplement to support your digestion of meat products, a vegetable based product is not your best choice. A vegetable based enzyme does not have the capacity to break down animal protein or fat properly making it an inefficient digestive aid for those who consume these foods.

A full spectrum comprehensive enzyme is recommended and the *Depke Wellness Prime Enzyme Support* contains both animal and plant based enzymes to replace the enzymes that are cooked out of your foods.

As a reminder, don't drink-water or other liquids 30 minutes prior to meals and 60 minutes after meals. Also, chew your foods thoroughly. These tips, along with taking a digestive enzyme, can help make a dramatic improvement in your digestion and improved bowel movements.

Stay Hydrated Between Meals

Being properly hydrated not only helps your fecal matter to move through the digestive system, it also helps in the formation of a healthy bowel movement. If you're dehydrated, the contents of your small intestines become solid and move very slowly into your colon. The contents of your colon absorb hydration via the colon walls, creating much more bulk, slowing movement even further. For healthy colon motility, follow the hydration tips discussed earlier in this book.

If you're not a water drinker, or feel it lacks flavor add a slice of fresh organic lemon, lime, or orange to your glass. Make an iced tea with herbal teas such as lemongrass, peppermint, or raspberry hibiscus. Be sure that the tea is herbal. Drinking caffeinated varieties such as green tea, white tea, or black tea, don't count as water intake, and are ultimately dehydrating. Enjoy herbal iced tea and make it a tasty addition to your daily hydration plans.

Move Your Body

To improve movement of your colon, increase movement of your entire body. My favorite method is to jump on a rebounder (mini trampoline) for about 10 minutes twice per day. This improves motility of the colon extremely well.

Squat Don't Sit

When you think of the toilet as a modern day convenience, you're probably pretty grateful, aren't you? Consider the ancient alternative: digging a hole, squatting over it, and then burying the entire mess. But, is this really an improvement? If you're like most people, you're probably unaware that the toilet is one of the worst designs for aiding in the process of proper bowel movements. Sitting upright on a toilet puts us in a posture that kinks your intestines, thus creating an impingement of the colon leading to troubled bowel movements.

We are naturally designed to squat.

You'll sigh with relief when I tell you that I'm not going to ask you to give up your toilet. There'll be no digging of holes. But I am going to ask you to raise your feet when using the toilet. I recommend using a small stool or any item that you can put your feet on to mimic the natural squatting position. This can be very helpful for most people.

There are also retail items designed specifically for this purpose. One product, The Squatty Potty®, tucks discretely around the base of your toilet and can be pulled out during use.

Release Your Emotional Stress and Baggage

Science has proven that stress, anxiety, and suppressed emotional trauma affect the body in many ways including slowing the motility of the colon. To simplify, on a physiological level, stress creates a sympathetic response (a "fight or flight" response). A relaxed state creates a parasympathetic response (a "rest and digest" response). This parasympathetic response increases motility of your colon whereas the fight or flight response slows it down.

The deep breathing exercises mentioned earlier can provide calming benefits, decrease your stress, and help the colon move. Refer to Chapter 7 in this book on *mental, emotional, spiritual, and energetic health.* There, you'll find great recommendations on how to release emotional stress.

Get Your Spine Aligned

Spinal alignment is also important to colon function. If you have misaligned vertebrae in the lower spine, this can impact your colon and affect motility. I have seen clients in the past who follow proper protocols to achieve healthy bowel movements, only to be derailed by a challenge in spinal alignment. Don't let this be you. It's worth investigating this problem with a quality local chiropractor.

Colon Hydrotherapy and Home Enemas

If you've ever been constipated at any time of your life, it's a good idea to look into hydro-therapy treatments or home enemas. I encourage both of these techniques as I've seen, firsthand, the positive impact they can have. I've seen these techniques restore health, aid in weight loss, increase energy, and detoxify health-challenged individuals. I recommend reaching out to a qualified colon hydro-therapist or a natural health practitioner who has a deeper understanding of the proper use of these treatments.

Acton Step:

Implement these steps, as they apply, into your daily routine. Put your smart phone to use and add daily reminders for anything you have a hard time remembering. Remind yourself to drink water, practice deep breathing, chew slowly, make herbal iced tea, raise your feet when going to the bathroom, get your body moving with exercise, and more.

Chapter Six

Exposure to the Sun

Haven't you been told for decades to stay out of the sun, cover up, and always use sunscreen? It's common knowledge that the sun's rays are damaging and dangerous, true?

No, this isn't true!

Exposure to the sun is an essential nutrient (yes, nutrient!) for our bodies. We need exposure not only through the skin, but through the eyes as well.

Most people only think about vitamin D in regard to sun exposure. The reality is that exposure to the sun has many additional benefits.

- Vitamin D is produced in your body via sun exposure
- Sun exposure releases endorphins creating an empowering mood and energy

- Sun exposure improves many skin conditions such as dermatitis, psoriasis, eczema, vitiligo and scleroderma
- Sun exposure was the accepted treatment for tuberculosis long before the introduction of antibiotics
- Healthy sun exposure is actually a protective measure against melanoma
- Sun exposure through the eyes significantly helps in the production of melatonin
- Sun exposure helps balance your natural rhythms of body and mind
- Sun exposure can decrease the pain of fibromyalgia
- Sun exposure helps prevent and reduce the symptoms of multiple sclerosis
- Sun exposure is essential to reverse seasonal affective disorder
- Sun exposure supports immune system function
- Sun exposure helps to regulate your core body temperature

Of course "healthy" sun exposure is the key. This varies for each individual because of the vast range of skin tones. However, a general guideline is to attempt about 30 minutes of direct sun exposure per day. If you have very fair skin you may want to limit this to less than 30 minutes and if you have a darker complexion, you may need more than 30 minutes daily.

The preferred time for peak conversion of vitamin D is between 11:30 am and 1:30 pm and interestingly, this is precisely when most of us have been told to avoid the sun.

Have you ever misjudged the time you've spent outdoors, ending up with skin as red as a lobster? Ouch. If so, you may recall your skin alternating with radiating heat and sudden chills. That, my friend, is extreme sun damage. Pay attention to the amount of time you spend in the sun.

Burns are to be avoided at all costs.

Be smart about protecting your skin. If you plan a beach day or a long day at the pool, take frequent breaks. Sit under a large umbrella and limit the amount of direct sun to skin exposure. If you are at a water park, wear a thin cover up that can get wet to protects your skin. In this case I'd also recommend using a natural non-toxic sunscreen.

On the days that you are getting adequate sun exposure, reveal as much of your skin as acceptable and avoid sunscreen or cover ups.

The more skin that's exposed, the higher the benefits.

If you react to sun exposure by developing rashes, this could be an immune system issue and should be brought to the attention of a qualified natural health practitioner.

We can't all live each day in a tropical paradise. If it gets cold and gloomy where you are in the winter, I highly recommend using a quality vitamin D supplement. Supplement each month of low sun exposure. Also, allow as much natural daylight to shine through your windows as possible during these months.

Another way to increase your vitamin D levels is to swap out your bulbs. Use a full spectrum desk lamp (if you spend time at a desk), and/or change the bulbs in your home to full spectrum. About 6 hours of full spectrum exposure is the equivalent of about 30 minutes of direct sunlight. Of course, natural sunlight is best, but when Mother Nature isn't cooperative, full spectrum lighting can be a great option.

Action Step:

Go for a 20-30 minute walk daily in the sun after lunch. This provides a triple benefit. You enjoy sun exposure, move your body moving and the walk will also help to stimulate proper digestion of your meal. That's a real win/win/win situation for you!

Chapter Seven

Mental, Emotional, Spiritual, and Energetic Health

This fundamental of health encompasses many things. Do you picture something different when you think of your mental and emotional health versus your spiritual health? And, what about your energetic health? Although these areas of your life are complex and vast, they beautifully intertwine with each other. They all have an enormous impact on your overall health, happiness, and your ability to heal. Some experts say these non-tangible states actually have the most significant impact on your potential to achieve wellness.

You are an emotional, spiritual, and energetic being. It's been said that we're spiritual beings having a physical experience.

Signs of a harmonious and balanced emotional state include, feeling fully expressed, healthy, happy energized, joyous, grounded, and connected. When this part of you is lacking, imbalanced or ignored, the opposite may be true. You may feel stress, sadness, frustration, and loneliness.

Your emotional, spiritual, and energetic self is a foundational part of your health and happiness. It's important to address any physical, mental, and emotional challenge you are currently dealing with. When you do, you will create a life overflowing with satisfaction, love, joy and happiness! If you're feeling depleted in these areas right now, you may not feel this is possible.

But I'm here for you.

I plan to empower, inspire, and educate you to a greater understanding.

Our Failing Health Care System

Here's a common scenario. A patient who feels completely stressed, lacking in motivation, unable to sleep and experiencing anxiety, goes to the doctor. Then what happens?

More often than not, the doctor diagnoses a chemical imbalance and an antidepressant or antianxiety drug is prescribed. There may also be a referral to a psychotherapist or psychiatrist. This road tends to lead down a rabbit hole of more pharmaceuticals and more specialists.

A drug or more drugs isn't answer. This approach fails to address the underlying causes of the stress, lack of motivation, sleep issue, and/or anxiety. The issues aren't resolved.

Perhaps this has happened to you? Maybe you've taken or are taking some of these medications:

- Celexa
- Lexapro
- Prozac
- Luvox
- Paxil
- Zoloft
- Pristiq
- Cymbalta
- Effexor
- Savella
- Fetzima

I might even agree, at times, with a doctor who suggests that there's a chemical imbalance but the reality is that people are not suffering from a deficiency Prozac, Paxil, Zoloft or any of the other drugs that are prescribed. There are specific short-term circumstances where these drugs may be useful, but they truly are not a long term answer. Let me show you why.

This subject could fill another book, so I'll keep it simple. Often, the imbalances mentioned above are directly tied into a number of factors. They may relate to our own perception of circumstances or experiences, a lack of communication, a lack of understanding, and/or a lack of knowing what natural treatments or protocols to use.

There are simple fast working techniques that can shift you from feeling stressed to feeling peaceful, or shift you from a place of frustration to a place of empowerment. It is truly amazing how fast lifelong issues can dissolve when focused action is taken. Although it's unlikely you'll hear of the following techniques from your doctor, I'm happy to reveal them to you.

Perception

Let's define perception. Perception is a way of regarding, understanding or interpreting something through the 5 senses. It's a way to form a mental impression. Have you ever witnessed a situation and then heard the person standing right next to you describe it differently? Why was their experience different? This is due to a person's personal perception. It's unique to each individual. It is the way a person experiences life through their five senses, memories, and past experiences. These influences have a direct impact on every circumstance they experience.

What if, for example, two people were each asked to describe the ocean? One might say it is majestic, beautiful, powerful, and brings a sense of peace. The other might say that it's scary and dangerous. Why so different? Let's add a bit of background. Perhaps the first person has surfed since childhood, finds comfort in the waves, and meditates on her surfboard. And, the second person had a near death experience in the ocean as a child. Do you see how their perceptions of the ocean would differ? Which one is right? Which one is wrong? This illustrates how we create our own unique perceptions of the world.

This is a very powerful concept. It can be life altering for those willing to look at situations from another's perception. Get curious. Ask questions when someone disagrees with you. Make an effort to understand their viewpoint and they may reciprocate. You're both right. No one is wrong. It's simply a matter of differing perceptions. Looking at life through someone else's viewpoint or perceptions broadens yours, too.

Have you ever heard the saying, "Nothing has meaning except the meaning you give it? The

131

result of this is a billion different meanings for each circumstance.

This makes the world a very interesting place.

Another area to explore regarding perception is what I call cause and effect reality. Are you at *cause* for your life, or are you living at the *effect* of your circumstances? Shifting from cause to effect can help you tap in to creating a powerful life regardless of what's happening around you. It takes a bit of practice, but self-empowerment comes from creating your life rather than being reactive to it.

Think to yourself, do you most often react to what others are doing or saying around you or do your create intentions to live into on a regular basis?

Reacting is living in the effect of others and creating is being at cause.

It's easy to fall victim to someone else's agenda, especially from "prickly people." If you can pause your knee-jerk reaction to their behavior, take a deep breath, and just observe them, you'll learn quite a bit. If they're overreacting or out of control, it's simply their unhealthy way of dealing with their own fears, thoughts, or perceptions. Yes, it's difficult if their comments are directed at you, but take an objective viewpoint. Is the "problem" theirs or yours?

The most important question to ask yourself is, what "healthy" action can you take?

Understanding your own position of objectivity empowers you in uncomfortable situations. With practice, these situations will impact you less.

There is significant freedom in no longer being at effect of others.

The next step in a confrontation is to acknowledging their anger or frustration immediately. Repeat their words. Let them know that you hear what they're saying. Then ask a few clarifying questions. Keep the questions short and to the point. By being at cause, and not getting sucked into the drama (becoming a victim), the other person naturally shifts from a defensive posture to one more open. This increases the opportunity for resolution and mended fences – both for today and tomorrow.

Another perception shift to embrace is the belief that everyone is simply doing their best with what they have. This means they're doing what they can taking these factors into consideration - how they were raised, their knowledge and personal skill set, what situations they have lived through, and their own choice of living at either cause or effect.

Of course, we don't always like another's "best." They probably aren't behaving as we think they should.

Of course, that judgement comes from our own perceptions, right?

But it is important that we accept their best, even if we don't agree.

People often misunderstand this principle of cause and effect. Accepting someone else's behavior isn't always the same thing as condoning it and that's not the intention. Accepting somebody's best is for your peace of mind – not necessarily theirs. Acceptance is the beginning of change for you. When you shift to a position of acceptance, compassion shows up in place of judgement.

Think of someone who lived through the Great Depression. They might judge you for buying an expensive handbag or car. From their perception (their sense of reality) your purchase is unnecessary, frivolous, and wasteful. Understanding how their perception was formed turns their judgement of you into a simple reflection of their own experience. This perspective allows you to separate yourself from their judgement. You instead feel compassion

135

for how their lack mentality has limited them in life. This position allows you to feel more in control, energetic and empowered.

I have learned to accept and have compassion for prickly people and/or those who sometimes demonstrate prickly behaviors. I know you can too.

Boundaries

You may be surprised to learn that setting boundaries actually creates freedom. Set boundaries for what you will or won't accept from the people in your life. Once boundaries are set, then you have a guideline for how you wish to be treated. There is nothing wrong with telling someone they've crossed that line.

When you practice acceptance and compassion, you'll notice that your boundaries are not crossed. You're living at cause for your life rather than at the effect of others.

Besides the emotional benefits, living at cause can play a significant role in calming your adrenal function. As your nervous system calms, you'll experience decreased stress and frustration. You'll shift toward a more accepting, loving, calm, and forgiving way of being.

If boundaries with others are new to you, here are a couple of examples.

- Your husband is a workaholic and you have personal needs that need to be met in your relationship. You can set a boundary that yourself and your husband have a "date night" once per week. This boundary would be discussed with your husband and you would set your date night. Now that the date night set and the boundary discussed, it is up to you to hold your spouse accountable to keeping this promise as well as yourself. If you let this slide and the date night doesn't happen, the boundary is worthless.

137

- You set a boundary nutritionally. Perhaps you chose to give up gluten and you are invited to dinner at a friend's house and this friend makes pasta and garlic bread, all containing gluten. While this may be uncomfortable to you, it is important to hold your boundary. Do not eat the gluten. Hopefully you will have an option of a salad or vegetable so this is not a complete loss. When you set boundaries such as this nutritionally, it is not a bad idea to mention your nutritional choices before agreeing to a dinner invite. Set yourself up for success, rather than failure.

Boundaries are only as good as your follow through. While these can at times be very uncomfortable, this truly sets you up in an empowering position.

Change Your Perception by Changing Your Vocabulary

Surprisingly, changing a few simple words or even just one word in your thought process can shift a stressful situation into an empowering one.

Here's a personal story that helps to illustrate this principle.

Years ago, I began working with a personal trainer. I must admit to dreading my workouts. I felt rushed and sometimes showed up late. My routine took place on Wednesdays after a very long workday. I noticed that every Wednesday afternoon toward the end of my day, I felt the stress and pressure of what I "had to do." My self-talk was negative (have to, got to, should, etc.). I was stuck in a "have to" mindset, creating unnecessary stress and frustration.

One day, I vividly recall feeling the "I have to..." thought in my head. I chose to make one simple

139

change. This change shifted my perception and my entire reality around this topic. I changed my thought of "I have to" to "I chose to." The thought of, "I have to go workout" became, "I chose to work out."

This was so much more empowering!

That simple change shifted my entire workout experience. I perceived it differently from then on. I realized that carefully choosing my words put me back in the driver's seat. I became at cause for my life and my choices. And, I enjoyed my workouts again.

Action Step:

Take 10-15 minutes and hand write your "have to" list. Once you have as many as you can think of, take a breath, and write down a few more. Write until you can think of no more. Next, cross off the words, "have to" and replace them with "I chose to." Feel the shift!

Not sure what I mean? Imagine saying, "I have to go to work." Go ahead and say it out loud. Now, shift that statement to, "I chose to go to work." Say that out loud. Sounds (and feels) different, doesn't it? Changing one simple word has great influence over how you think and feel.

Once this becomes second nature, you will find yourself noticing other words and thoughts that you wish to change. The impact of these shifts is far-reaching. As your perception shifts, your stress naturally decreases, your ability to forgive expands, and your ability to see another's position becomes easier. This new skill improves your inner thoughts and feelings of positivity.

Stress and the Impact on Your Mental, Emotional, Spiritual and Energetic health

I mentioned earlier that science has proven that stress, anxiety, and suppressed emotional trauma affect the body in many ways. We discussed how the motility of the colon is impacted. These situations also have tremendous effect on the mental, emotional, spiritual and energetic body.

It would be great to live a life of love, joy, happiness, abundance, confidence, and forgiveness all of the time, wouldn't it?

Sadly, many of us instead live a life filled with fear, guilt, anger, sadness, irritation, lack, and blame.

Would you be interested to learn how to shift out of this unhealthy paradigm?

I thought so!

Action Step:

Take a moment and honestly ask yourself which emotions and energy you experience most frequently. What do you feel on a daily basis? Is it fear, guilt, frustration, or lack? What about joy, happiness, confidence and forgiveness? Perhaps it's a combination. There is no right or wrong response. This is just an exercise to increase your awareness.

Let's discuss spiritual/energetic health for a moment. Some of you might automatically assume this refers to connection with a higher power and/or going to church. But I'm referring to a connection or action outside of you. Instead, I'm referring to your spiritual connection on the inside.

I work with clients from around the world and I am sure you can imagine how their opinion on this "energetic body" varies. Some call it vibrational, some spiritual; others express a combination of both. I've also heard many names used to describe the energetic body such as chi, qi, prana, vital force, life force, God, Buddha, Allah, Jesus Christ, Mother Nature, and the universe.

No matter the name, description, or belief, this spiritual connection is vital. This spiritual connection constantly moves through and within you.

This energy helps to keep you in the best of health.

This spiritual energy links directly to your emotions. For example, suppressing negative emotions creates a block in your energetic body. This blocked energy leads to disharmony, then dysfunction and ultimately leads to a physical health issue.

A state of dis-ease (a lack of ease) follows. Another way to define the word, "disease" is an imbalance within the energetic and emotional body.

This lack of energetic movement creates a stress response in the body. Remember the fight or flight response we discussed? When you are living in a constant state of fight or flight, the unhealthy cycle continues. You are stuck in this stress response creating a downward spiral in both your physical and emotional health.

The body CANNOT heal from the sympathetic fight or flight response. Healing begins within the parasympathetic response of rest and digest.

This is why proper energetic flow is vital.

Your adrenal (energy) glands and your sympathetic "fight or flight" nervous system are engaged when reacting to stress in your life and they react and interact with each other. Remember that any stress affects your adrenal hormones and your sympathetic nervous system. A long term reaction on this level leads to weight gain, fatigue and frustration and can be the beginning of any chronic illness.

Your nervous system is the master regulator of all function in your body. This is a powerful reason why working through your emotional baggage helps to get your body's energy flowing again. Once this happens, in no time you'll slip into your skinny jeans, have all of the energy you desire, and feel successful, fulfilled, and joyful.

Let me point out something you may have already have noticed: it's hard to see your own "stuff." When it comes to emotional baggage, it takes some detective work – ideally from an outside source – to help make things clear. If you feel that you have deeper mental or emotional challenges, I encourage you to seek the attention of a health professional.

For the everyday stress of life, here are some action steps that will shift your body into a healing rest and digest state. These techniques are sure to bring peace, comfort, and ease to your life.

Energy Tapping

Energy tapping, also known as Emotional Freedom Technique or EFT is a quick and effective way to help you reduce stress, anxiety, and move beyond suppressed emotional trauma. I use this both personally and professionally.

An abbreviated description of energy tapping includes tapping on particular head, facial, and torso acupressure points with your fingers while saying out loud the feeling/emotion that is being experienced. Tapping has been shown to shift someone in a very emotional state to a calm relaxed one in moments. This is a technique that you can use on your own once you understand how to do it or have working with a trained professional.

For more information as well as a detailed description of how to benefit from energy tapping visit www.emofree.com or www.DepkeWellness.com, Specialties link in the upper heading and click on Energetic or Emotional Release.

Deep Belly Breathing

You've noticed that I frequently reference deep belly breathing in this book, haven't you? This is such a powerful tool to help deal with stress and frustration.

Deep belly breathing can transition your body's response to stress from the sympathetic to the parasympathetic system. Make a regular practice of 3 – 5 deep belly breaths once per hour during your waking day. Additionally, use this empowering tool when you feel stress, anxiety or any other negatively charged emotional situation. Make deep belly breathing a habit. Deep belly breathing calms your nervous system, reduces cortisol production from your adrenal glands and allows you to take action with a sense of clarity. Gaining a sense of empowerment from deep breathing is good for both you and those around you.

Getting Back to Nature

When did you last lie in the grass and watch puffy clouds float by? Have you intentionally walked in the rain lately? How old were you the last time you dug your toes into wet mud, or warm sand?

We may enjoy the activities listed above, but don't make time for them. We jostle back and forth from our homes, to our workplace, restaurants, grocery stores, shopping malls and other buildings. We commute from place to place in traffic and our only outdoor time spent is walking across one parking lot or another.

This pattern wreaks havoc on our mental, emotional, spiritual, and energy body.

So, what is the solution?

Keep it simple. Get outside, get in the sun, and take a walk. Take time to connect with nature. Find a place that makes you feel a sense of joy simply by being there. Walk in the woods, walk along old train tracks, or walk on the beach. Your area of choice might be limited to your own neighborhood. That's fine, too. Notice the beauty nature has to offer right outside your front door. Remove your shoes and let your bare feet touch the earth to experience the positive healing benefits of grounding. Just walk barefoot in cold wet grass, soft soil, or warm sand.

Wintertime brings other outdoor adventures to light. Bundle up and take a walk enjoying the beauty of a recent snow fall and the freshness of the crisp air as you breathe. You may also enjoy outdoor winter sports such as snow shoeing, ice skating, skiing, or snowboarding.

Make it a priority to get outside every day. Breathe fresh air. Witness the beauty of the world around you and how you view your troubles will naturally come into a healthy perspective. Getting out into nature is a beautiful way to reconnect with your spiritual self.

Move Your Body

Moving your body has so many health advantages that the powerful stress relieving benefits it can provide might be overlooked. Exercise can be simple and should be something you enjoy. Telling yourself that you either do not have the time to exercise or that you are too tired demonstrates two glaring signs that you need to move your body.

Make it simple, fun, and consistent.

I totally understand. You may be over-scheduled and responsible to bosses, clients, family, friends, etc. We're pulled from all sides.

I get it!

Here's where I prescribe a mindset shift. Your health is just as important, if not more, than the rest of your responsibilities. After all, if you're not healthy enough to tackle what needs to get done, then who will?

Here's where being at cause can help.

You're in charge of your own health. No one sets boundaries around your "free time" schedule but you. If you're not taking empowered action regarding your own health goals, then now's the time.

Another fitness objection I hear often is, "I don't have the money." Exercise classes, gym memberships, and personal training can be pricey. If your budget does not allow these luxuries, then make another choice. Here is a list of free or low cost activities that can try today. Some are just as effective as and maybe even more fun than a gym membership.

- Walking
- Hiking
- Jumping jacks
- Bike riding

- Crunches
- Push ups
- Squats
- Playing sports with friends
- Tennis
- Swimming
- Rebounding
- Fitness classes in your local community center
- DVD for yoga or other fun types of exercise that is right for you

Think about what type of activities are fun to you. Jot down your ideas and expand upon this list. A lack of money is truly no roadblock to fitness success.

Is your level of fatigue out of control? This is typically tied into your adrenal health. More details about this important subject appear in the Bonus Section of this book. However, it's important to mention here that the right type of exercise actually helps your energy levels increase while healing your adrenal imbalance. On the flip side, remaining sedentary contributes to a worsening of your adrenal function. The key is to keep your exercise simple, easy, fun, and in bursts. (Refer to the *movement* section of this book and try different types of exercise such as walking or burst training. See what feels best to you.)

You don't need to commit to an extreme exercise program to gain benefits. Let that guilt go and don't make it complicated. Simply find what works for you and start now.

I also hear the complaint that fitness isn't fun. If you are pushing yourself to exercise and do not enjoy it, then it's not a long term solution for you.

Find something you enjoy.

Do bicep curls make you cringe? Do something else. Does running feel like punishment? Find an activity that puts fun into your fitness.

For example, I happen to like the outdoors. Rather than a gym routine, I'd rather play sports with others. Or do something such as walk my dog, go for a hike, go for a bike ride, play tennis, walk the golf course, or play a little basketball. While I do see a personal trainer in a gym twice per week, the majority of my fitness activities are outside, flexible, and enjoyable to me.

Working with a personal trainer provides support, challenge, encouragement, and accountability for me. If I wasn't held accountable to someone else, I'd probably be less committed to this part of my fitness plan.

Enjoyment is the key for long term success!

Prayer and/or Meditation

Prayer and meditation are two effective ways to reduce stress and both lead you to the rest and digest response of your nervous system. They will also help you connect with your spiritual self, your creative self, and your personal connection to a higher power, or the universe.

If you believe you've never meditated, you probably have, but didn't recognize it as meditation. Have you ever driven home from somewhere and not remembered some part of the drive? You likely dropped into a trance state which is much like meditation. If you have ever listened to music and your world of worries seemed to disappear for a time, you likely experienced a meditative state.

A meditative state is achieved when you allow yourself to slip from mental, conscious awareness into the present moment. The present moment alone consists of stillness and what I like to call "nothingness." It's a place of subconscious moments that center on peace and lightness.

Mediation does not have to be difficult. It can be as simple as sitting still and focusing on your breath for five minutes. When unhelpful or unwanted thoughts come into mind, simply let them flow and return to a focus on your breath. When this becomes easy for you, increase the time frame. The more you practice, the quieter your mind becomes.

You may also enjoy moving meditation. For example, walking alone in a forest with complete focus and appreciation for your surroundings allows your mind to become still. Some prefer connecting body movement to creating a calm mind.

If this is you, get moving out in nature by yourself and focus on your senses. Notice the different shades of green. Listen to the breeze rustle through the leaves. Enjoy the birds chirping or whatever beauty that speaks to your heart. Once your mind has quieted and your walking pace becomes trancelike, allow your mind to be still. From this level of meditation, you'll experience heightened creativity, intuition and gratitude.

Prayer is very powerful for helping us to feel connected to a higher power, a higher purpose, or to the universe. Prayer is another method of stress release and it's also a form of meditation as well.

Prayer has been scientifically documented to have a positive and significant impact the following areas of your life:

- Self-control
- Increases forgiveness
- Improves your outlook
- Increases trust
- Alleviates stress

All of these results from prayer have an optimistic and healthy impact on lowering stress levels in your life, increasing connectedness, and fostering a sense of belonging.

Tai-Chi Chung and Restorative Yoga

Tai-chi chung (or Qigong) and restorative types of yoga are two amazing tools to reduce stress. They both use the powerful combination of movement with deep breathing, and slow, concentrated movements. I highly recommend both of these for stress relief and for increasing the connection to your inner spiritual and emotional body. These effective practices generally require a qualified instructor to begin. Through practice, you may become confident enough in your form, posture, and methods to practice on your own. This knowledge can be handy as you may wish to practice in a park, the beach, or anywhere in nature.

Both yoga and tai-chi can be healing and beneficial for the whole body. But, don't forget about form and posture. If moves are done improperly (even slow moves), they can lead to discomfort and potential injury. Be sure to gain proper training before attempting on your own.

159

Attending a live class with a qualified instructor is ideal. But, if this is impractical, there are many CD's and online classes offering tai chi chung, or restorative, Iyengar, or yin yoga.

Share with Friends and Loved Ones

Do you recall the sense of relief you felt the last time you shared something heavy on your heart with your best friend? Good friends and loved ones know just what's needed when you feel down. They may offer advice, a laugh, or a hug.

I believe sharing has become a lost art. In many cases, it's been replaced by constant complaining. Simply sharing a stressful situation with a loved one can be powerfully beneficial for both of you. Sharing allows you to let go of the heavy emotional feeling tied to stress.

Some refrain from sharing because they confuse sharing with complaining. They don't want to appear to be a whiner. Here's the difference. A complainer wants no help, support, or even worse, advice. They only want agreement that their situation stinks. This is not the same thing as sharing.

We all have stressful situations in our lives and having someone serve as a sounding board can be very uplifting.

When sharing, be specific about why you are sharing and what you need them to do. You may just wish to get something off your chest, or perhaps you'd their input or advice. *Be very clear about your expectations.* Missing out on this step can lead to confusion and even hurt feelings. This can actually be more stressful in the end.

Sharing starts out in one of two ways. Here are suggestions to try:

- I have something that I would like to share with you and I really just need somebody to listen to me for a moment.

- I have something that I would like to share with you and I would love your input and advice on this if you'd be willing.

If you're clear in asking what you need in the beginning, you'll avoid frustration later. Sharing helps to divide our stress and after all, we are our best selves when in community.

Your mental, emotional, spiritual, and vibrational stress is at the foundation of all your fundamentals of health. To help your body release extra weight, the fatigue you're experiencing, and your frustrations, this is where to begin.

Stress is a primary factor that affects your adrenal health. Poor adrenal function leaves fat in your mid-section, some level of chronic fatigue, and a reduced ability to cope with stress. This can only leave you with high levels of frustration in your life. Look for further discussion on this topic in the Bonus section of this book.

Complaining, rather than sharing, can have the opposite result than you desire and actually add to your stress. Here's a simple rule of three's guideline to guarantee your success. Chose no more than 3 people to share your stressful situation with and that's it. This limitation has a healing effect and prevents the complaining trap.

Bonus Section

Deeper Healing

I touched upon how hormones play a role in your sleep cycles. However, they also play an important role in weight, energy, and stress reduction and management. They play such a crucial role in helping you to achieve the levels of health you desire, that further details are needed here.

Stress and Hormones

Stress comes in many forms. I invite you to contemplate for a moment, and really think about how stress shows up for you.

When you think of stress what comes to mind?

Perhaps it's work, unending responsibilities or little to no personal time. Under these conditions, it's common to make poor food choices despite having a healthy food plan. You tell yourself that convenience-wins over the quality of your food and this false belief may stand between your goals and what is preventing you from losing those nagging last 15 pounds.

Stress ties into so many areas of life beyond the mental and emotional stress just mentioned.

Stress may also be tied into:

- Illness (chronic, or reoccurring acute illness)
- Infection (primarily unknown infections in the gut)
- Injury (either recent or chronic)
- Inflammatory (bloating, aches and/or pain, etc.)
- Toxicity (exposure to silver amalgam fillings in your teeth, chemicals in foods or airborne, or simply living in our toxic environment)

It's good to investigate the impact these stressors have-on your body. Any level of stress pushes your body into a fight or flight response, thereby wreaking havoc on your adrenal (energy) glands. Your adrenal glands are the first responders to any and all levels of stress in your life on any and all levels.

I'll repeat that. Any level of stress, large or small, quick or long lasting, creates a response from your adrenal glands. You have two tiny triangular adrenal glands that sit above each kidney and play a powerful role in the function of your entire body.

They're tiny but mighty!

Do you feel that you've been stressed out for so long that you're skilled at handling it? I'm here to tell you that long term stress, of any kind, has a negative impact on these tiny energy glands. If the stress becomes chronic, and the adrenals aren't able to regulate that response, the damaging results become holistic.

Examples of these results are listed below:

- Weight gain
- Thyroid issues (insufficient energy)
- Sugar cravings
- PMS, menopause symptoms, or infertility
- Bloated belly
- Fat around the midsection of the body
- Food allergies or sensitivity
- Headaches
- Muscle or joint aches and pains
- Weak immune system
- Up and down energy levels
- Weakened bones
- Poor recovery from exercise
- Poor mental clarity
- Mood swings
- Inability to fall asleep easily
- Insomnia
- Feeling tired when you wake up (the snooze alarm is your best friend)
- Poor memory and/or concentration

Here is a chart that shows the impact of adrenal function on your body. The middle circle that reads "cortisol:DHEA ratio" is tied to your adrenal function and EVERY circle outside of the middle circle is dependent on healthy adrenal function.

This is the "ah...ha" moment for most of our clients.

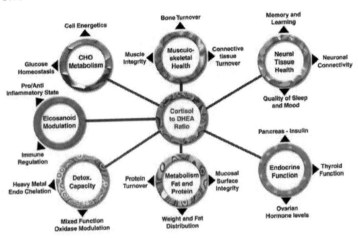

So ask yourself the following questions.

1) *How many of the above symptoms pertain to me?*
2) *What can I do?*

Perhaps you feel these symptoms are just a part of the "natural" aging process? I'm here to tell you, there's nothing natural about chronic health challenges. We've come to believe that watching sick people age (become sicker), is a part of the natural aging process.

The true natural aging process is to maintain a very high level of function and energy until nearing the end of life. Study any indigenous culture and you will find this to be true.

Do you feel as if you have no choice in the matter? Your life just runs on autopilot and you're along for the ride, right?

Take a deep breath. Let go of the struggle. You don't have to be stuck in this rat race forever. I have answers for you. I share what I've learned with others every day. I unlocked the mystery of great health for myself years ago.

I can tell you it's not only possible, it's within your reach! Follow the two important comprehensive steps below.

FIRST:

Implement the fundamentals of health as outlined in this book.

Congratulations for reading this far!

Go ahead and re-read all of the action steps listed in each chapter and create your own personal health a plan for you today.

The sooner you begin the sooner you will be in control of your health. In no time, you'll slip into those skinny jeans, wake up feeling refreshed, have sustained energy throughout the day, and feel happy, successful, proud and confident!

SECOND:

Get your adrenal (energy) glands working again. They're likely burned out from managing all of the different types and different levels of stress in your life.

All body functions are dependent on proper hormone balance. Specifically, adrenal gland function must be assessed and addressed.

A comprehensive adrenal gland test can be done very easily by collecting a small amount of your saliva 4 times within a day. I'll share with you how to get this simple kit below.

Here's an important fact. My team of experts and I have reviewed over five thousand adrenal gland tests results. And, of these, how many would you guess have shown a "healthy" result at the onset of a new client?

We have only seen five return with healthy and balanced adrenal function.

No, that was not a typo. I did say only FIVE! Why is that?

In fairness, we work with people like you, who have health challenges. So, it is safe to say people with a range from minor to major health challenges have issues with burned out, stressed out, tired adrenal glands. What we've discovered, is that *the combination of addressing adrenal stress coupled with implementing the fundamentals of health is where we see the greatest improvements*.

Here are action steps you can take immediately.

Action Steps:

- Take vitamin B5 – Every hormone produced in your body is dependent on this B vitamin. So, if you have a hormonal imbalance you are likely deficient in vitamin B5. We recommend the *Depke Wellness Prime Adrenal Support* for this.

- Pay attention to your mental and emotional response to stress. Start with awareness and then implement the action steps found in the section on *Stress and the impact on your mental, emotional, spiritual and energetic health.*

- Food sensitivity – Either test for food sensitivity with a holistic professional, or I recommend a helpful book on this subject, "The Plan" by Lyn-Genet Recitas.

- Reduce inflammation – This is a typical chronic trigger for most with adrenal issues. This is best done under the guidance of a qualified natural health care practitioner. In our wellness center, we address this through an on-line program called, The PAIN of Inflammation.

- Assess and address pathogens – Many people are living with unknown pathogens such as parasites, protozoa, detrimental bacteria, H-pylori infections, and more. Assessment requires the help of a qualified natural health care practitioner. In our wellness center, our preferred method to address this is via stool testing. Specifically via BioHealth Labs, the gold standard in the field, using a test kit number 401H.

- Toxicity – A toxic body strains the adrenal system. Focusing on your fundamentals of health along with balancing your adrenal function may be all the support you need. Some people have deeper toxicity challenges that may require testing and personalized detoxification protocols. I do not recommend detoxification programs until you have – at minimum addressed your fundamentals of health and improved your adrenal function. Detoxification is typically not a good starting point.

Addressing these areas is essential to for you to see results in your life. Following these directions will help you shift from feeling *fat, fatigued and frustrated* to feeling young again.

Find your lean, energetic and fulfilled self!

Another challenge tied into poor adrenal function is referred to as your HPA axis (your coping mechanism). The job of this coping mechanism is to drop your body into a deeper state of relaxation after a stressful event, situation or time frame in your life.

This is a natural occurrence and is necessary to restore balance after stress. This coping mechanism is the reason why many of us can endure high stress with some regularity, yet still maintain high levels of health and happiness. When the coping mechanism is working correctly, every time we have a stressful event, it engages and induces the body to feel a deep sense of relaxation.

It acts as our body's "reset button."

When this system is working properly, we *always* return to a balanced state, after stress.

The problem though, is that under constant stress, this coping mechanism can begin to burn out. When relentless stress occurs (instead of periodically dropping into a state of relaxation and balance) stress simply begins to accumulate.

When you see this pattern in your own life, you now have the power to do something about it. A telltale sign is small stressors you handled easily in the past now push you over the edge.

This is a loss of your coping mechanism and a breakdown of the HPA axis. Don't worry though; you can help your body rebuild this. In order to rebuild and repair it's necessary to address adrenal dysfunction. It plays a complex part of the entire HPA axis.

These systems need to function together in harmony.

There is no known laboratory test that can assess the level of health or dysfunction your HPA axis. However, adrenal function can be tested. From these results, we can create a completely individualized healing program for you.

Customized wellness leads to true healing at the deepest level.

Best Way to Test Adrenal Gland Function

Adrenal assessments may be done through either saliva or blood tests and I recommend using saliva testing. The accuracy of saliva testing allows you to see hormones that are built up or stored in the tissue of your body. You're also able to see the fluctuation of hormones over an entire day. Blood tests do not provide this information. They only show specific hormone levels at the specific time the blood was drawn. And, you're not able to see the levels of hormones stored in the tissue or body at all.

Shocking Case Studies

I had a client who was slightly overweight, fatigued, and completely frustrated with her health. She was working with a holistically minded medical doctor who suspected she had hormone imbalances and proceeded to test via blood. This blood test showed low progesterone levels, and concluded that this was at the core of her health problem. The doctor recommended she supplement with progesterone.

Sounds sensible, right?

After all, if something is low, you should supplement to increase the levels, shouldn't you? Unfortunately, when dealing with hormones it's not that simple. I wish it were, but it isn't.

Motivated to heal, this client religiously put on her new prescribed progesterone cream and was tested monthly to assess the effectiveness. Month after month the testing revealed that her progesterone level was only minimally increasing. So the dose was continuously increased.

After a long year with little change she felt hopeless. Upon finding my wellness center, Depke Wellness, we immediately tested her adrenal function and secondary hormones via saliva testing. After her yearlong protocol with increasing doses of progesterone cream, her saliva test revealed something very different than her blood test had shown.

Her progesterone level in her saliva was over 46,000, which was the highest level I had ever seen. The normal level of progesterone for this postmenopausal woman should have been between 5 and 95!

Astounding, isn't it?

Now, you're probably wondering why these levels registered in her saliva, but not in her blood? This is a great question.

Her absorption through the skin was poor. Absorption of hormones via skin has the potential to be very inconsistent, leaving a potential tremendous buildup of hormones in the skin and surrounding tissue. The vast majority of the prescribed hormones never made it into her bloodstream.

Think this is an isolated incident? This happens all of the time. It happens with both progesterone and estrogen creams. One alarming side note is that high levels of estrogen can cause estrogen dominant breast cancer.

Men are at risk, too.

I recall a male client who told his original doctor that he was fatigued, lacked motivation, and had a low sex drive. The doctor ordered a blood test for testosterone and found his level was low. He was prescribed testosterone pellets to be surgically implanted into his arm. They would slowly release testosterone into his body over the course of 6 months.

When we took him on as a client we ordered saliva testing for his hormone levels. Upon review, we found something that many would find shocking. His testosterone levels were low but his estradiol was through the roof! His estradiol hormone should have been between 1 and 3 for a male, yet it was above 13.

Just as elevated estrogen hormones are a risk factor for women and breast cancer; high estradiol is a risk factor for prostate cancer in men.

I have helped countess people over the years recover from improperly monitored use of hormone creams. It's become a passion of mine. It's fascinating and rewarding to create customized health programs for people who that have lost hope ... and see them heal.

The joy of these customized health programs is that they initiate the body's inherited ability to heal. You are stimulating your natural healing process.

It's an art and science, combined with years of experience, which allows my team and me to look at hormones and make sense of the puzzle. We review hormones such as progesterone, estrogen, cortisol, DHEA estradiol, estriol, testosterone, androstenedione and melatonin and assess your current state of balance.

It has taken me years to master this protocol and teach my team.

I would love to not only give you hope, but serve as a catalyst for your complete healing. I'd love to help you find the happy, healthy, confident you again.

The First Step to Assessing Your Adrenal Health

Now that we know how intertwined the systems of the body are, it is now time to assess your adrenal and hormones function levels.

Because you are already experiencing some health challenges, it's likely that your hormone health has been imbalanced for some time. This is true even if your symptoms have just begun. Next you'll find an easy assessment for your convenience. Take it now to determine your current state of adrenal health.

Adrenal Stress Profile Assessment

Next to each question assign a number between 0 and 5. Assign values as follows:

0 = Not true 3 = Somewhat true 5 = Very true

Once you have completed the questionnaire calculate your total and locate your score.

	I experience problems falling asleep.
	I experience problems staying asleep.
	I frequently experience a second wind (high energy) late at night.
	I have energy highs and lows throughout the day.
	I feel tired all the time.
	I need caffeine (coffee, tea, cola, etc.) to get going in the morning.
	I usually go to bed after 10 pm.
	I frequently get less than 8 hours of sleep per night.

	I am easily fatigued.
	Things I used to enjoy seem like a chore lately.
	My sex drive is lower than it used to be.
	I suffer from depression, or have recently been experiencing feelings of depression such as sadness, or loss of motivation.
	If I skip meals I feel low energy or foggy and disoriented.
	My ability to handle stress has decreased.
	I find that I am easily irritated or upset.
	I have had one or more stressful major life events. (ie: divorce, death of a loved one, job loss, new baby, new job)
	I tend to overwork with little time for play or relaxation for extended periods of time.
	I crave sweets.
	I frequently skip meals or eat sporadically.
	I am experiencing increased physical complaints such as muscle aches, headaches, or more frequent illnesses.

Scoring Your Adrenal Stress Profile:

It is important to note that this is not a diagnostic test and should not be used to diagnose, cure, or treat any conditions. It is simply a tool to help assess your potential level of adrenal insufficiency.

If you scored between:

0 – 30   You are likely in good health.

31 – 40   You are likely under some stress.

41 - 50   You are likely a candidate for adrenal burnout.

51 – 60   You are likely in adrenal burnout.

61 +   You are likely in severe adrenal burnout.

*Special thanks to Dr. Daniel Kalish at KalishInstitute.com for the use of this adrenal assessment.

So what was your score?

I've created a summary of information for each scoring range. Look for your specific health range below.

If you have scored between 0 – 30

Congratulations! I'm very excited for you because you are most likely already enjoying some very positive health practices that I would encourage you to continue. Be sure you implement many of the components of the fundamentals of health that will take your health to the next level. And, I'll say congratulations again. Most people in our stressed out culture do not meet this score!

If you have scored from 31 – 40

You are likely under some stress and this is already beginning to affect your adrenal function. If you find yourself in this area I would recommend that you review the fundamentals of health found in this book, and determine which are lacking for you. It is a good idea to consider taking a Vitamin B5 supplement to support all your adrenal stress hormones. In my office I recommend a form of Vitamin B5 referred to as Pantothenic Acid. I've seen positive results with a dosage of one 500mg capsule daily. The combination of addressing your fundamentals of health and Pantothenic Acid support can assist your body in getting back into balance.

If your score totaled between 41 and 50

It is recommended to test your adrenal function with the saliva testing. This is a good place to catch your adrenal imbalance. At this stage, it's not likely to have caused many deeper health issues, yet. But, if left unaddressed, a path of health challenges may await.

To test adrenal function, I recommend working with a qualified natural health care practitioner. This working relationship isn't just for proper testing but also to create an ongoing game plan to assist you in balancing this function. I would recommend working with a practitioner that is certified in either the Kalish Method or the Depke Method of adrenal balancing. My team of experts work with people from all over the world and more information can be found at DepkeWellness.com.

If you scored between 51 and 60

You are likely in adrenal burnout and probably have other health issues that are fueled by long term adrenal hormone imbalance.

As mentioned in the information for a score range of 41 and 50, I recommend working with a qualified natural health care practitioner. My recommendations are to work with a practitioner that is certified in either the Kalish Method or the Depke Method of adrenal balancing. My team of experts work with people from all over the World and more information can be found at DepkeWellness.com.

You will most likely have additional challenges to address in reaching your ultimate health goals. But what you've learned here will set you on the right path for yourself.

If you scored a 61 or above

I would address this in the same fashion mentioned in the score levels above. And do not delay. This is likely a deeper issue for you that needs attention and balance.

This potential level of extreme adrenal burnout is most likely affecting you in many ways. Please address this level as soon as possible.

I'm so happy and grateful now that you have begun implementing the fundamentals of health as outlined in this book. You're following the action steps and finding your own levels of health success. You are creating new healthy habits that are in alignment with the new fabulous you.

Here's what else I see for you now that you've completed this book and have taken action.

You not only can easily slip into your skinny jeans, but everything you put on looks great! Your levels of energy have increased, and you enjoy drinking plenty of water between meals. It's easy to make healthy food choices and you find that getting out into nature is rejuvenating for you. You're connecting better with friends and you feel successful at everything you do. A new confidence has sprung forth and your happiness is evident. You hear people telling you everywhere you go that you look young and vibrant and they want your secret.

This life is possible. I see this type of transformation all of the time.

You're ready to make the changes you need, aren't you?

Enjoy the process of creating the life of your desires!

Thank you for your dedication to a lean and energetic body and a life of ease. For further information on health feel free to visit DepkeWellness.com.

Made in the USA
Monee, IL
25 July 2020